THE SEA GLASS EPIDEMIC

THE SEA GLASS EPIDEMIC

JODI LYONS

Rand-Smith Books

The Sea Glass Epidemic

Copyright © 2024 by Jodi Lyons

Print ISBN: 978-1-950544-43-1
Digital ISBN: 978-1-950544-44-8

All rights reserved. No part of this book may be reproduced in any manner whatsoever without written permission except in the case of brief quotations embodied in critical articles and reviews.

Rand-Smith Books
www.RandSmithBooks.com
USA

First Printing, 2024

This is a work of fiction. Names, stories, characters, businesses, and events are anecdotes for illustrative purposes only. Any resemblance to actual persons, living or dead, is purely coincidental.

While this story offers insights into a medical condition, it is intended for informational purposes only and should not be taken as professional medical advice.

Contents

Prologue		1
1	JANUARY - EVERYTHING IS NOT AS IT SEEMS	3
2	FEBRUARY - COMING HOME, AKA RECOVERING FROM A VACATION	12
3	MARCH - IS THERE A ZOMBIE APOCALYPSE COMING?	29
4	APRIL - PREPARING FOR THE APOCALYPSE	37
5	MAY - SPRINGTIME DURING THE APOCALYPSE	45
6	JUNE - IS IT A NIGHTMARE OR REALITY?	68
7	JULY - THE MOUSE ARRIVES	80
8	AUGUST - THE POLTERGEIST IS MERCILESS	87
9	SEPTEMBER - ROSH HASHANAH, THE START OF A NEW YEAR	94
10	OCTOBER - THE TRAVEL BUG HITS	98
11	NOVEMBER - THANKSGIVING	109
12	DECEMBER - THE DESCENT	128
13	JANUARY – THE LANDING	138
14	FEBRUARY – THE CRASH	154
EPILOGUE		157

notes — 161

Acknowledgements — 162
About The Author — 163

Prologue

Could the Bermuda Triangle have engulfed Washington, D.C.? To some, the Triangle is a portal to another place; to others, it's nothing more than someone else's hallucination. Usually, it's thought of as a place of mystery, fantasies, dreams, and nightmares. Often, it's the backdrop for science fiction stories. What if other places, like New York, Las Vegas, or Washington, D.C., held the same mystery as the Bermuda Triangle? Or, what if the forces behind the Bermuda Triangle traveled with individual people?

What powers the Bermuda Triangle? Where did it come from, and what is it? Is it caused by a meteor? Is it a wormhole? Is it designed by aliens? Is it a zombie gateway? Whatever the origin, structure, or purpose, clearly, whatever was behind the Bermuda Triangle was taking over Washington, D.C. Something strange was going on. It was particularly curious, however, that not everyone seemed to be aware of something bizarre happening.

Can some people sense things other people can't, like a canary in a coal mine does? If something is real to a particular person and no one else can see it, hear it, or smell it, is it still real? Where's the line between imagination and hallucination? Dreams and reality? Belief and delusion? Faith and science?

Beth, an avid traveler, was feeling rather philosophical as she pondered the case for a meteor, a wormhole, or relocation of the Bermuda Triangle to explain the oddness in Washington, D.C. As she pondered, she stood in her bedroom in a D.C. suburb and halfheartedly packed her clothes for yet another business trip. Wistfully, she hoped something exciting might happen on this one. Beautiful, but it was quite boring. The most exciting thing that happened was that her banana was confiscated at the airport before she had time to eat it prior to boarding her flight home. Apparently, her intended breakfast had violated some agricultural rule. She had a nagging feeling in the back of her mind that this trip was going to be different. For a fleeting minute, she hoped for an encounter with a meteor or a wormhole, anything to make this trip less boring. She'd been woefully disappointed with her trip to Bermuda and her lack of encountering anything Bermuda Triangle-like. She decided the nagging feeling in the back of her mind was wishful thinking and put it out of her head.

"Same old, same old," she thought to herself. "Another day. Another trip." The big fat bear lounging on the chair in her bedroom disagreed. He was an annoying bear. He sat there in all his multicolored rotund glory, taking up the entire chair, so she had no place to sit down when she was putting on her shoes. He grew fatter by the day. And, sometimes, he would shed onto the floor. His primary diet was clean laundry. Most people understand that doing laundry is a pain in the neck; people tend to leave it in the washing machine, forget it, rewash it, and finally move it to the dryer. Eventually, the laundry makes it to a chair, usually in a bedroom. But putting the clean laundry away seems to be an insurmountable chore. There are internet memes making fun of this process. Beth's laundry chair is occupied by a bear fortified by clean laundry. His size and scope rival the mythical laundry mountain. Beth talks to him regularly. Sometimes, he even answers her.

Today, the bear was amused by Beth's haphazard packing. She usually was better than this. He could tell something was different. This time, she was indecisive about what she was packing and kept packing and unpacking the suitcase. Idly, he wondered if she knew something was different. The thought was short-lived, however. He became distracted by unmatching all her socks in the pile and hiding a select few. He found it funny. It was a trick he learned from the dryer.

Eventually, Beth finished packing, zipped the suitcase closed, and put it by the front door so she'd be ready to catch her flight in the morning. She sighed as she got ready for bed, already anticipating her flight. At least it was a nonstop. Her travel agent apparently had had difficulty finding one from Baltimore to Las Vegas.

I

JANUARY - EVERYTHING IS NOT AS IT SEEMS

Las Vegas is hot. It may seem like an obvious statement, considering it is in the middle of the desert, but for Beth, a native New Englander, the heat struck her like a tidal wave. That's probably a terrible analogy because the desert is arid. A tidal wave would have been welcome. At least it would have had some moisture in it. The air was so dry it made her skin hurt. She remembered her friends who had moved to Las Vegas had told her the heat wasn't that bad because it was "a dry heat." She knows they are either delusional or lying to her. It is ridiculously hot. Every time the airport door to the outside opened, Beth was subjected to a blast of hot, dry air as if she were standing in front of an exceptionally large hairdryer.

As she stood at the baggage carousel waiting for her luggage, Beth felt every minute of her fifty-seven years of age. She used to be a road warrior, traveling hundreds of thousands of miles per year and never paying attention to the trials and tribulations. As a matter of fact, she used to be one of those people who got annoyed at the tourists who were not moving quickly enough through the airport, took too much luggage with them, couldn't find their seats, and, in general, had gotten in her way. Recently, however, she's slowed down, both physically and mentally. Maybe it's normal aging. Or it's sheer exhaustion. She prefers to believe she has become more tolerant as she ages. She did nothing more than blink when, while boarding their flight, her seatmate banged her in the head and stepped on her toe while trying to fit an enormous duffel bag in the overhead bin. But standing at the baggage carousel, she reflected on how uncharacteristically mellow she was. Normally, she'd never check a bag. Why would you have to wait an extra fifteen minutes for your luggage when you could carry it yourself and race out of the airport while everyone else is waiting for their bags? That way, you could be first in line for a taxi or hotel shuttle.

This time was different, though. Beth was exhausted even before she got to the airport and fell asleep on the flight. That was unusual for her. She had been complaining for decades that she was completely incapable of sleeping on a flight, no matter how long it was. That led to some entirely miserable red-eye flights. This time, she "conked out" almost immediately. Since she was so tired when she got to the airport for the beginning of her flight, she decided to check her bag instead of lugging it with her. While normally she was quite good at juggling her roll-aboard suitcase, her laptop case/pocketbook, and her lunch, which she inevitably grabs at an airport restaurant before boarding the plane, she didn't have the energy this time.

Nor did she have the patience to deal with what she was sure would be a planeload of tourists. You know the type: they carry far too much luggage which they try to fit in an overhead bin when there's no way it will, they can't find their seats, they take forever to move down the aisle, and they take even longer to deplane. They also are the ones who gather in front of the jetway door, eagerly awaiting their seat row to be called for boarding, and in the process, they manage to block the door for everyone else who is trying to board. In general, they are annoying for road warriors who travel all the time, especially those who have status to pre-board.

For this particular flight, however, Beth admitted defeat before it even happened. She knew she wasn't up to traveling in her usual road-warrior manner. So, she minimized the stress on herself. As she stood waiting for her baggage on the carousel, she remembered why she never checked her bags. The fifteen minutes she expected to wait turned into half an hour. And, inevitably, she found herself standing next to the tourists who obviously didn't think their never-going-to-fit-in-the-overhead-bin-luggage was enough and had checked additional bags.

At least their behavior was consistent. Instead of blocking the door to get on the plane, they were blocking the carousel so no one else could get their luggage. She wondered what they knew that she didn't that required so much luggage. She can travel for a week in her 21-inch roll-aboard suitcase. She traveled with the basics that could be mixed and matched to create multiple outfits. That, and a few changes of accessories, were all she needed to give two or three presentations, attend a few receptions, and even sneak in a bit of relaxation time at the casino. For her to carry a full-sized suitcase like they did, she'd need to stay for a month. Maybe that's what they were planning.

She was so wrapped up in trying to understand the behavior of the swarm of tourists surrounding her with their millions of pounds of luggage that she never noticed the tall, slender, rather nondescript man standing next to her. He was puzzled by the behavior of the people around him. It was even more than that. He was intently observing their behavior as if he were analyzing it. Had Beth noticed, she might have found it unusual or even spooky. She definitely would have noticed he seemed inappropriately dressed for the weather. He was wearing jeans and a heavy, bulky blue sweater. Again, it was hot in Vegas. But Beth didn't notice him. That also was strange for her. She usually was much more aware of her surroundings.

Still pondering what could possibly be in the huge amount of luggage the tourists were carrying, she settled into a taxi and headed to the convention center. She was surprised to see a line of taxis outside the baggage claim area. Normally, in this day and age, particularly since she wasn't first off the plane, she would have assumed there weren't going to be any taxis left, and she would have called the rideshare service. But since she was lucky, and the taxi already was there, it seemed easier to hop into the taxi.

As they drove away, Beth was a bit surprised she hadn't noticed the man sitting beside her in the backseat. She nodded hello to him and then checked her messages on her phone. He was entirely silent and completely motionless. The driver pointed out some tourist sites along the way, and Beth answered him, but the silent man remained silent. Beth thought it a bit rude, but she also thought she might be being a bit hypocritical. After all, she had her nose in her phone while she was talking to the driver. When they got to the convention center, the driver got out to help Beth remove her bags from the trunk. Beth looked back into the backseat, and to her surprise, the silent man no longer was there. "That's strange," she thought. But the thought was fleeting. She had other things to do.

Once she paid the taxi driver and handed her bags to the bellhop, she snapped into convention mode and followed the same routine every road warrior follows... She picked up her conference registration packet, went to the hotel registration desk, got her room key, and went to her room to unpack and verify her schedule. The hotel room was gorgeous. It was clean, modern, and hot. Apparently, this fancy new hotel had energy-saving devices that raised the room temperature when the system sensed an empty room. It seemed as though hot and dry-as-a-desert was the theme of this business trip. Sarcastically, she thought to herself, "I can't wait till I'm sitting under the hot lights on the stage for ninety minutes giving a presentation! That'll feel great." She decided to rethink her presentation outfit. Typically, convention center meeting rooms are freezing, even for a Bostonian like her. She had packed accordingly, but this time, "freezing" could be relative to the outside temperature and therefore still would be hot. It's so much harder for women to dress for presentations. The men have it easy. They change their tie and take off their blazer, and they still look totally professional. They are fine regardless of the temperature. Women usually can't get away with taking off their blazers and having a tank top underneath while doing a presentation. Fortunately, Beth had enough options in her small suitcase to cover all eventualities. She was a pro, after all.

Feeling confident in the hotel's security, Beth unpacked her laptop and put it out on the desk instead of leaving it in the in-room safe as she normally would. She logged in and let it boot up as she stored the case in the bottom of the closet. Recently, she's been careful about not leaving things on the floor, even something like a laptop case, because she's been losing her balance, and she was trying to minimize her risk of tripping. As she was standing with her head in the closet, putting the laptop case away, she swore she heard voices coming from her room. It puzzled her for a second, but then she brushed it off. She's had far too many experiences with Siri on one device talking to Siri on another device. They can have some funny conversations as one version of Siri tries to make sense of what the other one is saying. Besides, this hotel was extremely high-tech. She would not have been surprised if the room itself was talking to one of her devices.

Having successfully stored the laptop case, she returned to her computer and checked her emails. Much to her delight, she realized she still had an extra ninety minutes before that evening's reception. Making good on a promise she made to herself decades ago, she went downstairs, opened the door to the hotel, and walked outside. The intention was to do something, anything, outside the hotel/convention center. She had spent far too many years being sequestered in hotels and convention centers in beautiful cities and never seeing anything outside of the hotel, convention center, or airport. So, she promised herself that at least once per day, she would open the door of the building, go outside, breathe some fresh air, and occasionally even leave the convention center grounds.

That was her plan today. She was going to take a look around the Las Vegas Strip. Until she opened the door and stepped outside, that is. It was freaking hot ("wicked hot," as a proper Bostonian would say). She turned around and went back inside. Then she realized there was a small casino in the hotel. She promptly lost twenty-five dollars at the roulette table because she didn't read the sign carefully and didn't recognize that it was a twenty-five-dollar minimum bet. That was her gambling money for the weekend. So, she wandered around the hotel, watching other people gamble. Then, she discovered the penny slots. That was more than enough to meet her needs. She enjoyed watching the lights flash, the wheels spin, and the colors change, like a mindless TV show with no plot or a less-than-challenging video game.

She dug through her purse for pennies. She found none. She forgot she had emptied the change out of her pocketbook before she left her house. She always cleaned her pocketbook before she went to an airport; no need for the TSA agents to dig through her crumpled-up tissues, old hard candy, receipts, multiple types of makeup, and loose change. Sighing, she took a dollar bill out of her wallet and put it into the penny slot. She certainly wasn't going to get rich, but at least she could keep herself entertained inexpensively — as opposed to the twenty-five dollars for one minute's worth of entertainment at the roulette wheel. She was bored within ten minutes. But, she was up three dollars. So she printed the receipt from the machine showing her credit and returned to her room.

Her lack of attention span and her apathy were a bit concerning. Something seemed off. Looking back on the day so far, she realized she had been totally mellow, for the most part, dealing with tourists on the airplane, checking a bag, sleeping on the airplane, and having the attention span of a flea. In general, she was lethargic. She realized she had made a rash decision about not exploring the Vegas Strip. Even though it was hot, she could have hired a car or gone on a tour bus. She didn't need to walk the whole Strip. And, a few minutes of gambling wasn't taking advantage of her surroundings. But, she didn't care. Realizing she still had an hour before her reception, she decided to take a short nap. Unfortunately, the stupid air conditioning had reset itself, and it was hot in the room. So, she lowered the temperature to "stun" and waited for the room to cool off so she could sleep. Thankfully, she settled into a deep, restful, dreamless sleep. It was an excellent nap, even if it was short.

The conference reception that night was beautiful. It was on the rooftop of the hotel and overlooked the Las Vegas Strip. The Strip at night is fascinating, even from the top of a remarkably high hotel. For Beth, it was as fascinating as watching the slot machine wheels spin. There were lights, lasers, music, and probably other things she couldn't see from her rooftop reception. Fortunately, the people were nice, the food excellent, and she felt perkier than she had the rest of the day. The earlier malaise was gone. It was a great way to start the conference. For a brief minute, she thought she saw and felt freezing fog. Freezing fog is an unusual phenomenon; it's a strange sensation. It's a fine mist, like regular fog, except it is bitter cold and feels like needles made from ice pellets. Standing on the roof deck of a hotel in a desert was not where one would expect to find freezing fog. But Beth was sure she had experienced it. She chalked it up to an odd occurrence and promptly forgot about it. She had a good reason for forgetting about the fog immediately… On the roof deck, directly next to her left foot, was a small stone, about the size of a nickel. It was round and smooth, concave at the top, and would make a phenomenal worry stone. When she picked it up, it looked like it was made from clear sea glass. She had no idea how a piece of sea glass ended up at a rooftop reception in a desert, but she thought it was interesting and put it in her pocket.

Fast forwarding through the rest of the rather uneventful conference, overall, Beth was pleased. The receptions went well, her wardrobe choices worked out fine, and she even managed to get in some time playing poker with her colleague. She kept making a funny slip-up, though, referring to the poker game as "har gao," which is a type of shrimp dumpling (and one of her favorites) instead of "pai gow," which is a type of poker. It struck her as odd, but she laughed it off and decided she was craving dim sum.

The trip home was too eventful, however. Her colleague had taken the flight home that departed ninety minutes before her flight. His flight took off fine. As she went to verify her flight time, she found out it had been canceled. Her flight was scheduled to be on an airplane type that had crashed a few times, and the aircraft had been taken out of service. There was no flight rescheduled.

She was mildly annoyed at this. Her normal response would have been to go ballistic at the lack of communication, to scream "agent, human, representative, moron" at the phone tree for the airline's voicemail, and to push random numbers on the phone to get to a human instead of being stuck in phone tree hell, all while trying to navigate the airline's app, and eventually resorting to sending flaming tweets about how incompetency of the airline. That always got an immediate response when all other attempts failed. It certainly was not that she was upset about their taking the plane out of service; rather, it was their lack of communication in not telling her the flight had been canceled even though the airline had her phone number, her email, her text, and she had installed the app on her phone. It surprised her that she did not yell, scream, or offer to reorganize the airline by firing everyone who did not do their job — her normal reaction when faced with incompetence. Of course, she did have a list of complaints. Clearly, the airline knew in advance they were not allowed to fly this particular aircraft; it had been grounded by the FAA for months. Obviously, the airline should have made other arrangements in advance. And, the airlines knew where to find her and the other passengers. There was no excuse for the lack of communication.

Surprisingly, though, she kept her list of complaints to herself. She was annoyed the airline had not informed her in enough time to get on the earlier plane with her colleague. But since this particular flight had been booked through a travel agency, she called them and explained she needed to get back somewhere near the Washington, D.C. area. They did, and they even were able to change her car service to pick her up at a new airport. Again, she was surprised at her apathy about this. Normally, she would have been miffed. But, she didn't care. She was not particularly pleased that it meant she got home at one o'clock in the morning instead of eight p.m. the night before, but she couldn't muster enough energy to get worked up about it.

A few weeks after her return from Las Vegas, she had a completely uneventful flight to Florida to visit her parents. This time, before she booked the flight, she did check to see what type of airplane was scheduled. While she wasn't perturbed particularly by the previous misadventure, she decided not to repeat it.

Something changed for Beth on that flight home from Florida. For some reason, she could not get a song out of her head. Multiple times a day, when she wasn't distracted by the TV or music playing in the background, and she thought she was going to get some quiet time, she'd start hearing the song "Something's Coming" from *West Side Story*. She was puzzled. It wasn't one of her favorite songs. She hadn't heard it on TV. It didn't come through any of her streaming music stations. It wasn't on her car radio. She was used to hearing TV commercials replaying inside of her head, but that was the purpose of advertising, wasn't it? This was different.

Beth hoped the song would foreshadow her social life's improving, winning the lottery, meeting Mr. Right, or something equally as positive and exciting. It gave her hope. She was wrong. It wasn't hopeful. It was the beginning of the end.

2

FEBRUARY - COMING HOME, AKA RECOVERING FROM A VACATION

It was a bright, sunny, cold February day as the airplane from Florida landed at the Washington, D.C. airport. As always, Beth smiled as she caught sight of the Washington Monument as the plane settled in on its final approach for landing. In the thirty-five years since she moved from New England to Washington, D.C., she had seen many changes, including the newly renovated airport at which she was landing, but the never-changing view upon landing and takeoff always reminded her of why she was here. It was, every pun intended, monumental.

Beth had moved to D.C. in her mid-twenties for graduate school. In her heart of hearts, she knew she never would leave. She was drawn to the city, the politics, and the overall vibe. Her family knew she was never coming home even before she did. She'd moved three times in her thirty-five years in D.C. First in an apartment, then into a condo, and now in a house. She always had worked in politics, or at the least, politics-adjacent, since arriving in D.C. Now, she was a lobbyist.

It was easy to forget that Washington, D.C. often operates within its own bubble. It's not unusual to have a traffic jam caused by a presidential motorcade, for example. People living in the nation's capital often feel they are living in a fishbowl, and someone is always watching. The local news is international news. That certainly was not the case in Florida, where she had been visiting her parents. There, the local news was local. The traffic jams were nothing compared to even the everyday traffic in the D.C. area. The dress code was much more casual, and the speed at which people went about their daily business was a significantly slower pace than Beth was used to in D.C.

Beth had plenty of time to ponder the differences between Florida and D.C. as she sat in the back of the rideshare car which was, as expected, completely stuck in traffic on the GW Parkway. Then, the car sat in traffic on the Beltway and Route 270. It was a two-hour flight on the plane and an hour and fifteen minutes sitting in traffic for what should have been a 25-minute ride. In any other city, that is. Washington, D.C., was notorious for its horrible traffic.

As was typical in a Washington, D.C., traffic jam, people weren't paying attention to what was happening around them. They were on the phone, using a hands-free device, of course, listening to podcasts, or listening to the radio. They paid as much attention as was necessary to avoid hitting the cars around them. The joke had been that one could land a spaceship in the middle of the D.C. Beltway, and people would honk if it traveled too slowly down the lane. But, they would never notice it was a spaceship. This was true today. If anyone had bothered to look, they would have noticed the vehicle in the middle lane looked like an old-fashioned airstream silver mobile home, but it had no tires and was hovering along the roadway. Caught up in their own worlds, the drivers never paid attention. Coming out of the back exhaust pipe was a fog-like mist leaving a sheen on the roadway behind it. It glistened in the sunlight and looked like black ice. Traffic was so bad that the cars rolling over the black ice melted it. Again, no one paid attention. They concentrated on fighting the traffic and getting home or wherever they were headed. Couldn't they see what Beth saw?

Once she returned home, Beth breathed a sigh of relief. She loved her house. It was small, about 1400 square feet, with a postage stamp-sized lawn, but it was in a wonderful neighborhood. Most of D.C. seems to be socially transitional, with people moving in and out with each change in presidential administration. There are career federal employees who stay put in certain areas, but there usually is a lot of movement in other neighborhoods. That means in many areas, neighbors don't know each other. They meet each other during natural disasters like the derecho windstorm or a blizzard, during security crises like September 11, or during "normal" neighborhood problems like the sprinkler pipes freezing in a condo and flooding out multiple units. Beth's current neighborhood was different. When she moved in, her neighbors came over to introduce themselves, and many brought homemade baked goods. It was so unusual from her prior experience in the D.C. area that she ended up calling friends and telling them. Most of them thought she was exaggerating. The look and feel of the neighborhood hearkened back to another era, or at least, to a different part of the country. It truly was a neighborhood, not quite as idyllic as the 1950s, but as close to a neighborhood where people knew each other and kept an eye out for each other as she had seen since she moved to D.C.

She was glad to be home. It was wonderful visiting her parents, and she truly had a fun and relaxing vacation. But, for some reason, she felt completely exhausted. She was so tired, in fact, that she stumbled while dragging her suitcase from the garage into the kitchen, even though there was only a tiny step. Cursing herself for not paying better attention, she felt lucky she was able to grab onto the built-in bookcase near the doorway in the kitchen to steady herself. She was glad it was a stumble instead of a fall.

As she settled in, she breathed a sigh of relief. Her house was filled with sunlight, the plants had survived her vacation, and the orchids in the sunroom had started to bloom. Too tired to unpack, she changed from her traveling clothes into sweats and ordered a pizza. That was it for the night.

The next morning, as she went to get breakfast, she realized she absolutely, positively had to go to the grocery store or at least order grocery delivery. Since she hadn't prepared a shopping list, she figured it was easier to go to the store, wander up and down the aisles, and pick up what she needed. Fortunately, she was a consultant, so her hours were flexible. "Flexible," in D.C. terms, means there is no break between home and work. So, she usually ended up working seven days a week. However, she had the "luxury of flexibility" and could go to the grocery store in the middle of the week in the middle of the day when it usually is less crowded than on the weekend.

It was the end of February, and Passover was in early April. Since she usually hosted two Passover Seders with twenty or more people at each, she always prepared months in advance. It made sense to pick up the nonperishable or freezable Passover food while she was at the grocery store today. Grabbing a fiber bar and a Diet Coke® on her way out the door, the breakfast of champions and her personal favorite, she decided to go to the large grocery store farther away that always had a wonderful Passover selection. It wasn't the most efficient choice since she drove past two other stores of the same chain on the way, but they never had the selection she wanted.

Fragments of a song ran through her mind. "Something's coming, hmm, hmm, hmm." Beth smiled to herself as she pulled into the parking lot. She wished she could remember the rest of the lyrics or know what the "something coming" was. Maybe she was going to meet Mr. Right in the grocery store. She had heard of stranger things.

For some reason, the parking lot was incredibly full, which was surprising given Beth's midday-midweek-avoid-the-crowds strategy. Since she already was there, she decided to go into the store and take her chances. Grabbing one of the large shopping carts proved to be a challenge since the store seemed to be out of large shopping carts and only had small ones available. That wasn't going to work for a pre-Passover haul. But she persevered and succeeded in finding the full-sized cart, thanks to her professional shopper/parking lot "shark" skills. She girded herself to face the crowds, strapped her pocketbook across her body, and elbowed her way into the store, which was complete and utter pandemonium. The store was ransacked, people were pushing and shoving, and there were big empty gaps on the shelves where products should have been. It looked like people were preparing for a hurricane or blizzard, but Beth hadn't seen anything about it on the news. Could this be why she kept hearing the song "Something's Coming" in her mind? She'd always focused on the "something good" part of the song, but maybe it was the pre-rumble part she should have been listening to... The people around her certainly were acting like something bad was coming. She decided to get in and out of the store as quickly as possible.

So, she headed over to the produce section, grabbed a few items, and then went to the Passover section. She loaded her cart with huge quantities of shelf-stable food she would not eat unless it was Passover. Feeding fifty people takes a lot of food. But, for Passover in particular, many of the food items are specific to the holiday and not something one would use during the rest of the year.

She loaded the larger items on the bottom rack of the cart, organized the inside of the cart as best she could, and then moved on to the dairy aisle. This was where she noticed a vast difference. There weren't all that many people in the Passover section, and the shelves were well-stocked. This was not the case in the dairy section. She was looking to replenish the staples that were standard for anyone who was returning from vacation: milk, eggs, butter, cream cheese, cottage cheese, etc. The grocery store employees were restocking the eggs since there were none on the shelves, so she was able to get some of them off the pallet. She had wanted whipped butter and sticks of butter, but they were out of the sticks. Fortunately, she grabbed some whipped butter. They were completely out of all types of cream cheese, yet there was plenty of cottage cheese. It seemed strange with what was available and what wasn't. For example, there was no cookie dough or sticks of butter, but there was plenty of yogurt. She was puzzled, but she was able to get almost everything she needed, even though it was different brands or types and much higher prices than she expected.

As she continued around the outside sections of the store, she was at the deli counter waiting her turn when she looked to her left and up the center aisles of the store. It looked as if people were getting into fistfights. It was interesting; there was nobody in the organic/natural aisles but a logjam at the chips and snacks section. She got her deli, went to the bakery to get fresh bread, and then made the mistake of going down the soda aisle. It looked like they were giving away soda. Her first thought was there must be an incredible sale on soda, and she should most definitely stock up. The soda availability was sparse, and people were pushing and shoving and using their carts to block other people's access to the shelves.

    Beth was always up for combat shopping. She loved the thrill of after-Christmas sales and the challenge of getting the best deals. She was most certainly not above using her cart to block someone else's access to get the items she wanted. It was the Boston-driver method of shopping cart etiquette. So, she headed into the fray. Normally, Diet Coke® is her drink of choice. There was indeed a sale on soda: three cases of twelve cans each for twelve dollars. Her thought was to get six cases. It was a good thought but completely impossible. There weren't six cases of Diet Coke® on the shelves. She figured they might have put it on an endcap since it was on sale, so she wasn't particularly worried. But, just in case, she decided to get cases of other kinds of soda. It wasn't going to go bad, and she could always use it for Passover. She was not particularly strict about whether the soda was kosher for Passover or not. As she reached to get cases off the shelf, a tall, thin, rather nondescript man wearing jeans and a bulky blue sweater reached around her to grab soda. He seemed to have eight arms since he was reaching and grabbing so quickly around her and taking so many cases from multiple directions. It stunned her enough that she did a double-take to see how many arms he had. She was sure she had seen a flurry of arms around her. But, she blinked, and realized he had two hands. Unnerved by what she thought she saw, she took a deep breath and grabbed whatever diet soda she could find. Her working theory was that it's not hoarding if she would use it in a reasonable amount of time. There's a fine line between being prudent and hoarding. She was right on that line.

    Walking down a few more aisles, she saw a display of large bottles of Coke® and Diet Coke® with the yellow cap and Hebrew written on the top of the cap. She had scored! A little-known secret is that the yellow cap signifies the Kosher for Passover product. Kosher for Passover Coca-Cola® is made with real sugar, similar to Mexican Coca-Cola. For those people of a certain age, it is the "Real Coke®." It's the one Beth and her peers grew up with before soda companies used corn syrup and other sweeteners. It was a special treat for Beth's friends. She'd been known to serve it at the Seders and use it as prizes, special gifts, bribes, and more for her friends. She once did a drive-by drop-off at her friend's office so he could drink his Passover Coke® in peace without having to share with his family. She'd used it as a bribe to reward friends who helped her move furniture. In short, this was an outstanding find. And it's not hoarding if you're going to use it, right?! She hurriedly rearranged her cart, all the while looking over her shoulder for the man with many arms so he couldn't reach around her and grab any of what she needed.

Then, she looked down the aisle in front of her. Her intention had been to buy a few cases of seltzer for the Seder. It seemed logical since she had started the whole Passover soda process. Determinedly, she focused on the left side of the aisle. She loaded the cases of one-liter bottles into the cart, which was getting incredibly heavy, and glanced over to the right side of the aisle where the bottled water usually was. The shelves were completely empty. It looked like the grocery store staff had emptied the shelves in order to replace the shelving units. There were signs and store tags below where the water was supposed to be, but not a single bottle on the shelves. Beth was puzzled, but since she didn't need bottled water, she wasn't all that concerned.

As she continued through the store, she noticed that pretty much everyone had cases of water in their carts. Puzzling, she thought, but she had other things she needed to get, so she concentrated on finding those items. She self-righteously skipped the chips and snacks aisle but noticed it was incredibly congested with a melee of shopping carts. She made a mental note of items she thought she could use from Costco, like disposable aluminum pans, foil, freezer bags, etc., and skipped those aisles. She figured she'd get toilet paper at Costco.

While she didn't need thirty-six rolls, she probably would need them after having fifty people in her house. But since she didn't want to head to a second store today, she figured she'd pick up a six-pack while she was standing in the grocery store. The shelves were completely empty, even of the kind no one likes but buys out of desperation; carts were scattered every which way in the aisle, and people were yelling and on the verge of rioting. Beth wouldn't even walk down the rest of the aisle. It was too scary. As she turned around to leave the aisle, she saw a store employee with a pallet full of toilet paper. He was handing out one six-pack at a time to each customer. So she took it, not giving it any more thought, and left.

She skipped the frozen food sections entirely because they were incredibly crowded and because she needed to make more room in her freezer to fit Passover food when she started cooking. Then she got to the checkout. The lines reminded her of the weekend before Thanksgiving, with every checkout line open and long lines of customers at each. It was, as she would say, "crazy busy." And the people were rude. People with overflowing carts were trying to go through the ten items or fewer lines because they didn't want to stand in the longer lines. There were people arguing and complaining about how slow the person in front of them was or how slow the cashier was, as if they themselves were much more important and much busier than anyone else. It was as if all social niceties had left the grocery store.

As Beth lifted her items onto the conveyor belt, her right arm and hand glitched. For a brief second, her arm felt like dead weight, and her hand wouldn't respond to what she wanted them to do. Then her hand started shaking. She attributed it to lifting the heavy cases of seltzer off of the cart and onto the belt. She should have paid more attention to the sign that said, "Leave heavy items in cart."

As she pushed her cart across the parking lot and unloaded it into the trunk, she thought more about her shopping experience. She hadn't been to this particular store in almost a year, and she wondered whether what she saw regarding empty shelves and nasty customers was typical for that store or something else was going on. She decided it had been such a thoroughly unpleasant experience that she was not going there again. It wasn't worth the tumult. And worse, she didn't get everything she needed. Worse still, she felt overwhelmed and exhausted, and there was no way she could make herself head out to Costco.

As she returned the cart to the front of the store, she saw something glistening in the sunlight. She bent down to take a look and found another piece of sea glass, the same size as the one she found in Vegas, but this time it was seafoam green. It was round, smooth, and concave on the top. She was puzzled about how sea glass ended up in the parking lot of a grocery store nowhere near the ocean. But she picked it up, put it in her pocket, and continued on her way. She felt a distinctive tingle in her fingers, upper arm, and into her head as she fidgeted with the glass in her pocket. It made her a bit dizzy, but she was getting in the car anyway, so she didn't think too much of it.

Too tired to do any more shopping, she turned on the radio and headed home. As she arrived, she heard ...*stores across the area are reporting food short*—before she turned off the car. "I'll say there are shortages," she thought as she began to unpack the perishable and frozen groceries. Then, she threw in a load of laundry, and sat down at her computer to begin working. Even though she had tried to keep up with emails while she was on vacation, there still were a few hundred which needed attention. And then there was the list of phone calls to return. Day one after vacation. She already was exhausted.

That night, as was her habit, Beth relaxed in bed and scrolled through her multiple social media accounts. It seemed as though not many of her friends had anything particularly interesting going on. It was the usual: posting pictures of their kids because of a challenge put forward to post ten pictures of their high school kids in ten days, other people posting images with a specific color in them because of yet another challenge, and lots of photos of food. Apparently, many people have lots of time to cook gourmet meals. Beth was envious. She was lucky if she had time to eat cold leftover pizza out of the fridge while she was working.

Out of sheer boredom, she looked at the helpful suggestions of "people you may know." She never knew any of them. With nothing better to do and tired of seeing the same people she didn't know over and over, she clicked "remove" to clear out the feed. And then, a funny thing happened. She started getting friend requests from people she didn't know, who didn't necessarily know anyone she knew, and she couldn't figure out the connection.

The photos looked benign enough — mostly tall men with brown hair standing in front of interesting backdrops: the Las Vegas Strip, a desert, New York's Times Square, the Golden Gate Bridge, the White House, and other touristy spots. They all had rather generic names like Jim, Bob, Dave, and typical nondescript last names like Smith and Jones. Most of the profiles were rather new, were established within the past six months, and had nothing more than updated photos and no real posts. She thought it was interesting they had reached out to her, and she was flattered. So, she accepted all of the friend requests. By the time she went to bed, she had five new friends, all of them single men and all of them chose her out of all of the other people on Facebook. As soon as she accepted their friend requests, they sent her messages saying how beautiful she was. She fell asleep that night with a big smile on her face.

She was pleasantly surprised when awakening well-rested the next morning. For almost a year, she had been a terrible sleeper. While she never had been a particularly good sleeper, usually averaging about five hours of sleep a night, in the past year, no matter how much time she spent in bed, she always was tired and often had trouble getting motivated. This night was different. She slept through the whole night and didn't wake up until her alarm went off eight hours later. Her whole perspective was different that next morning. She was alert, productive, and tremendously focused. She was thrilled when she managed to bang out three columns for client newsletters: one that was due that day and two to "keep in the hopper" for future days when she had writer's block. She was "on her game." It felt good. She hadn't felt this way in a long time.

It was amazing what a good night's sleep could do. In addition to writing three columns, Beth finally unpacked from her trip, did her laundry (although she did not put it away and instead threw it on the chair in her bedroom), put away the rest of her groceries, cleared out her email box, and miracle of miracles, even vacuumed the floor. It made sense for her to take advantage of her burst of energy. It had been almost a year since she'd felt this good. That night, as she was getting ready for bed, she felt a sense of positive anticipation. Maybe tonight, she wouldn't toss and turn. Maybe tonight she would once again sleep through the night.

Of course, Beth was not that lucky. Two nights in a row of good sleep was not going to happen for her. This night, everything was back to her annoying usual night's sleep. She was hot, then she was cold. She had leg cramps that got better when she would kick her legs around or get up to walk. When she did fall asleep, her dreams were bizarre, nightmarish, and lifelike. She'd inevitably wake up in the middle of the night, drenched in sweat, and start pacing. That would start the inescapable cycle that had become Beth's life. She was so tired during the day she would often sleep for three hours in the middle of the day, zone out when she should be doing something else, and be cranky and unmotivated. Then, she'd still be exhausted at bedtime but couldn't sleep well. Over the past few months, she had developed a particularly strange habit; strange even in the context of the other weird things going on in her life, she would stare at the TV set for an hour or more as if she were watching a TV show. The problem was that the TV wasn't on. She didn't seem to notice or care. Idly, as she paced around the living room, Beth wondered if she had seasonal affective disorder.

February, in general, was a pathetic month. Beth was zoned out, apathetic, and exhausted; the weather mimicked her mood. It was cold and gray. There wasn't even any beautiful snow to brighten things up. Instead, February was nothing more than the dirty, gray, semi-melted dregs of snow left by the snowplows in the parking lots: dirty, played out, useless, and an eyesore. There was slush, mud, and ice everywhere. The gray sky and the gray dirty ground were indistinguishable from each other. It's a good thing that February is the shortest month of the year. The worst part is February is far too early in the year to be looking forward to spring. So Beth "hibernated" for the rest of the month. She couldn't get motivated to do anything.

Her house and her housekeeping reflected her lack of motivation. Dirty laundry piled up, dirty dishes piled up in the sink, she hadn't made her bed in more than a month, the floor was in desperate need of another vacuuming, the unread newspapers and magazines piled up around the house, the bathroom needed a good scrubbing, and there were crumbs on the kitchen counter. Beth didn't care. Since the weather was so gross, people were not visiting each other, anyway, so it probably didn't matter much. However, it was out of character for her.

Worse yet, the song "Something's Coming" kept running through her mind. But she didn't care. That also was unusual and out of character for her. Beth liked to be prepared for every eventuality. She always had "coffee and..." Meaning, she always had coffee and something sweet in case somebody dropped by. She always had something quick to whip up for dinner in case somebody dropped by. Her house was always clean in case somebody dropped by. She always was prepared in case something bad happened, like the power went out, or the freezer broke, or something like that. And, since she lived alone, she always had whatever medicine or first-aid kit she might need in case she got sick or hurt and there was nobody there to help her. Odds were good she already was prepared for the something that might be coming; it was unusual for her to not care about it. Yet, the song still haunted her.

Her dreams haunted her as well. Usually, Beth thought her dreams would help her work out something that was bothering her. For example, her best ideas for columns or strategic plans came to her in the middle of the night. She'd written excellent webinars and presentations at five o'clock in the morning after being woken up by dreams that guided those presentations. But these dreams were different. The most vivid she could recall was toward the end of February. She was in a strange house. It was a huge house, more like a mansion than a house. It was decorated in that fussy, overdone, nouveau-riche-pretending-to-be-regal style that Beth hated. Velvet everything and fake gold-plated everything dominated the full marble columns and floors throughout the house. Worse yet, everything was obviously faked to look old even though it clearly was bought within the past few years. Fake antiques were everywhere, and Beth was certain she recognized the "antique, distressed, real wood table" as one she'd seen at the self-assemble furniture store for ninety-nine dollars. Clearly, someone had stained it and distressed it by smashing it with cans, as she had seen on one of the DIY TV shows. In the first part of her dream, she was walking through the house as if she were a prospective homebuyer. She noted the layout of the rooms, tried to identify which potential changes were cosmetic versus those that were structural, and, in general, enjoyed exploring even though she found the design of the house completely atrocious. She decided the structure of the house was okay, even though everything inside of it was clearly fake. It was like being on the set of a cheap movie. "Maybe it photographed better than it looked in real life," she thought to herself.

Then, she walked into the kitchen and gaped in amazement. It was stunning, a professional chef's dream. It was enormous, had real marble countertops, a huge island with a ton of storage space, a sink in the middle, an indoor grill, and a baking center built-in with plenty of room for rolling out cookies, kneading bread, etc. It even had a full-sized oven built into the island, and a commercial stand mixer next to the island. Beth's favorite feature, however, was the pullout drawers in the island that housed commercial-sized containers of flour, sugar, and all of the other bulky baking things that no home ever has the space for.

On the other side of the kitchen was a commercial oven and stovetop. It was a 48-inch, natural gas, eight-burner stovetop with a double oven. It was exquisite. Above it was a special faucet tall enough to fill a giant lobster pot with water. Beth could envision her giant commercial stock pots on the top of this stove quite easily. Turning her head, she saw that the oversized sink was close enough to the oven so she would be able to lift the enormous stock pots to drain into the sink, and the sink was big enough for her to wash them in. She was smitten. Across the room, she discovered the commercial-sized refrigerator and freezer. The butler's pantry, in addition to having enough room to store all of her crystal and China and entertaining dishes, had a full-sized beverage refrigerator, a dishwasher designed especially for delicate glassware, a second dishwasher designed for huge serving platters, and a commercial ice maker. The walk-in pantry was the size of most people's bedrooms in a normal house. Much to her delight, the shelves were designed to hold large items like big boxes of cereal, family-sized bags of chips, Costco–sized cases of soda, and giant cans of tomato sauce. It was the kitchen set-up of Beth's dreams, and the house had the entertaining space to match. Sighing to herself and wrapping herself tighter in her covers, Beth happily dreamed about what the house could look like if she stripped off the ugly wallpaper, the fake gold, and the velvet.

It was then that her dream turned into a nightmare.

She felt like someone was watching her. Even though all of the lights were on in the entire house, all of the fireplaces had roaring fires in them, and the rooms were uncomfortably bright, Beth felt darkness descending on her. As she walked through the rooms faster and faster, she grew colder and colder. It was as if she was growing colder from the inside out. She understood the term "bone-chilling" cold. She felt something following her. She turned around and saw nothing was there even though she could feel something was. She knew she had to flee, to escape, to get out. It was as if the soul of the house was deeply insulted that she hated its decor and wanted to capture and harm her.

She walked faster, trying to find her way out. Instead of finding an exit, she ended up going bedroom to bedroom, en suite bathroom to en suite bathroom, hallway to hallway, never finding a stairway down or an exit out. She heard a whirring noise, and all of the shades in the house went down and covered the windows. The lighting in the house switched to nighttime mode and grew dimmer. Music, which she assumed was supposed to be soothing, came out of unseen speakers. She heard voices: "entering nighttime mode," "dimming lights," "starting music," "you can ask me to play specific music," "tomorrow's weather will be 34° with a 40% chance of sleet in the morning," "setting coffee maker for tomorrow morning," "would you like me to set up a new routine?" That was the last straw for Beth. The disembodied voice followed her from room to room, turning lights on and off, talking to her, and she couldn't escape it.

The house was so huge that no matter how fast she ran, she still was stuck in the endless supply of bedrooms and bathrooms and hallways. The feeling someone was watching her, and the sound of the disembodied voice were relentless. Faster and faster, she ran until she found a walk-in closet. She thought she could hide there and escape from the thing following her and the disembodied voice. So she ran into the closet and slammed the door shut. It was at that moment, she realized there weren't any locks on the closet door and whatever was following her could open the door, and she would be trapped. Taking her chances, she flung open the door, saw nothing looking for an escape route. She checked the next bedroom door she saw and realized there were no locks on it, either. All of the locks were fake. They were decorative, they looked like they should have keys, and there were no keys anywhere to lock or unlock the doors.

Faster and faster she ran, growing more and more panicked, and still she couldn't find a way out. The disembodied voices called out louder and louder: "You asked me to remind you to set the oven to 350°. Do you want me to set the oven now?" "Telling faucet to fill dog bowl with 32 ounces of water." Beth had no idea who had reminded this disembodied voice to set an oven. Was someone in the house with her? Was that person following her? Worse yet, she couldn't even find the oven and was afraid the house could catch on fire if this disembodied voice did set it and no one else was in the house. She was comforted by the thought that there might be a dog in the house. Otherwise, why would the disembodied voice be talking to the faucet and asking it to fill a dog bowl? As Beth continued to run throughout the house, searching for a way to escape, she became more and more certain someone or something was watching her. The lights would turn on automatically when she entered a room and turn off as soon as she exited. The hallway lights would turn on in front of her and turn off behind her, so at no time were all of the hallway lights on for her to get oriented about where she was or where she was going. And that disembodied voice talked to her through the ceiling and the walls. It always seemed to be right near her. She was beyond terrified. There was no escape.

To make things worse, Beth realized she had to go to the bathroom. She recalled seeing thousands of bathrooms as she raced around trying to find an escape. Yet now that she needed one, she couldn't find an acceptable one. The first one she came to had no toilet. The second one she came to was under construction and it looked like the toilet was disconnected. The third one she came to was filthy.

Beth stopped her panic-stricken running briefly because that last bathroom stunned her. Everything else about the house was in poor taste, in her opinion, but even so, it was immaculately clean. She couldn't figure out what was wrong with that bathroom and why it was so filthy. But, it was unusable, and now she needed to find a bathroom. So she stopped wondering about it and started running again. The next bathroom she came to looked like the communal stalls one would find in a rest stop on the side of a major highway. The stalls were small, the toilets were child-sized and too low for any normal-sized adult to use, and they were filthy. As Beth looked even closer, she realized that none of the stalls had doors, and the room was filled with strangers, all of whom seemed to be looking at her. Desperate to use the bathroom, Beth decided she had no choice and started to remove her pants to use the toilet in front of everybody. It was at that moment that she woke up. She realized she was safe in her bed, alone in her house, totally tangled in her sheets and blankets, covered in sweat, and needed to go to the bathroom. She called out, "Alexa, turn bedroom light on," and the light turned on. "Alexa, turn bathroom light on," and the bathroom light turned on. "Would you like me to turn the living room lights on?" Alexa asked helpfully. "No, thank you," Beth answered politely. She never knew why she said please and thank you to Alexa, but habits of a lifetime were difficult to break.

As Beth finished using the bathroom, straightened her sheets, and got back into bed, Alexa turned off the lights and adjusted the temperature in the room to be the optimal 68°, Beth's preferred temperature for sleeping. Still disoriented from her nightmare, Beth turned on the TV to try to relax a bit before she went back to sleep. Listening to the weather report for the upcoming week, Beth decided February sucked.

Things were made worse when she was writing her last column of the month. She had made a large pot of pumpkin spice coffee. Yes, Beth loved pumpkin spice anything. But, pumpkin spice coffee was her favorite. She bought dozens of one-pot-sized packets every fall and used them throughout the winter. This day was the day of the last packet. She filled her giant insulated mug with coffee made exactly how she liked it and then realized she couldn't find the lid. So, although on some level she knew better, she brought the giant mug of coffee sans lid and put it on a coaster on her desk next to the computer. Of course, the predictable thing happened. She spilled the coffee. Fortunately, most of it spilled on the desk, and since her computer was on a raised rack, the computer itself was not damaged. However, Beth managed to spill a mug of hot coffee on her lap. "The perfect end to February," Beth thought to herself. What else should she expect from a dreary, muddy, cold, gray month in which she had over 250 spam calls about her car warranty?

3

MARCH - IS THERE A ZOMBIE APOCALYPSE COMING?

February finally ended, and March rolled around. Something big was coming. The signs were everywhere. Beth still couldn't get the *West Side Story* song out of her head. What exactly that something was — was a bit unclear, but the signs were everywhere. She no longer thought it was something good. Would it be a zombie apocalypse? An alien invasion? Both? A meteor? The Bermuda Triangle spreading to Washington, D.C.? Retribution from life on other planets for our space junk circling the earth? It had to be something like that. There had to be a reason, something big, to make so many people act so strangely. Apparently, she had missed the first sign when she was at the grocery store six weeks ago. Absentmindedly, she fidgeted with the two pieces of sea glass she had put on her coffee table.

Scrolling through social media, she noticed some of her neighbors were asking if anyone else had seen a big, round, green light, something similar to a meteor, flying through the air near Washington, D.C. at one o'clock in the morning. Many people claimed to have seen it, and some claimed to have heard it. Beth was disappointed she hadn't seen or heard it. Much to her surprise, she didn't see anything in the newspaper, online (outside of social media), or on TV.

Beth had started obsessively watching TV. Perhaps it is more correct to say Beth kept the TV on constantly and would stare at it mindlessly. The TV news reporters urged people to avoid crowds and told them they'd be better off staying in their houses. Apparently, there was some zombie infestation in China that could come to the United States. From what Beth could gather, the contagion spread quickly, and no one knew how it spread, but it was dangerous. Once infected, people acted strangely and turned into zombies. They still looked vaguely humanoid, but they behaved differently, and it seemed as though this behavior spread among friends and family. Every news channel obsessed with this story. Some said it was an alien influenza brought back to Earth by the astronauts at the international space station, while others said it was nothing like the flu. Some said it was a disease brought back to life when the polar ice caps melted due to global warming. Others said it was a plague that had killed the dinosaurs and was reactivated when the fossils were dug up. Some said it was the rising of the undead ahead of the messianic age. Others said it was bioterrorism. Still others said it was political and the zombies were taking over the world. Then, of course, there was the debate over whether it was the zombies people should be worried about.

Nobody had clear guidance on what people were supposed to do, so people either were panicking as if a hurricane or a blizzard was coming, denying there was any problem coming, or doing their best to be prepared. Even as preparation levels were debated and implemented everywhere on TV and on social media, it was exceedingly clear the zombies were coming, or worse yet, they already were here, and they were taking over the planet. Nobody ever accurately described a zombie. Technically, everyone knows the word zombie means somebody who is undead. But it also seemed to be the type of term that applies to anything we as humans didn't understand, like aliens versus zombies. Identifying if either or both were real and knowing which was good and which was bad should have been "a thing," but it wasn't. The talking heads in social media were so busy debating zombie versus alien theories in the context of the Bermuda Triangle, the Egyptian pyramids, defrosted woolly mammoths, and possible Martian encounters that people were drawn into the debate, and nobody noticed the faceless, rather nondescript "people" moving into neighborhoods around the world. Even more confusing was none of the meteorologists seemed to be puzzled by small pockets of freezing fog in major cities around the world. If one looked, one could see the airplane contrails throughout the sky looked different and shimmered more than usual before the mist drifted down from the sky. Beth wondered whether this was related to the green light in the sky. She quickly was distracted from that thought, however, by yet another news report of fistfights in stores when it wasn't even Black Friday sales. She was puzzled by the pandemonium in the stores and the extent to which it was detailed on the news.

People who lived in a hurricane or blizzard territory knew what to do in natural emergencies. They made sure to have batteries, flashlights, canned food, and other things like that. Having grown up in Boston and survived the blizzard of 1978, Beth was surprised at some of the items people hoarded. Bottled water, for example. She guessed it made sense during hurricanes when the power could go out and flooding could interfere with the ability to get clean water, but she wasn't quite sure how that related to zombies. Also, she wondered about the toilet paper situation. Don't people normally have toilet paper in their house? Why were they grabbing seventy-two rolls at a time? What were they going to do with it? She was just old enough to remember "TP-ing" the trees in front of people's houses on Halloween, but it was nowhere near Halloween. And, an average-sized family had to take months to use seventy-two rolls of toilet paper, and that would assume they had none in the house before they bought seventy-two rolls. The news reports, in addition to covering the strange, zombie-inducing infestation, featured many stories of grocery stores with empty shelves and people waiting in long lines to be handed one 16-pack of toilet paper and one case of bottled water. It was as if the whole country was at war, and people were afraid of rationing even though that had not happened in the United States since World War II.

Most confusing of all was the not-completely-explained relationship between China and zombies in the United States. Beth liked Chinese food, so she was concerned it may be killing people. Or, at the very least, turning people into zombies. The news and social media reports were describing a zombie apocalypse. A lot of people argued on TV about how one becomes a zombie or who/what is killed by Chinese food. Beth didn't quite understand any of it. It didn't make any logical sense, and the stories were disrupted by a lot of yelling, accusations of people lying, people questioning whether or not there are zombies, arguments about whether the zombies are fed by a virus or hatched by aliens, and a lot of blaming other people. It was challenging to understand and got even more confusing when people yelled about Chinese food while they were boycotting Vietnamese and Korean restaurants. In fact, it was virtually impossible to make sense of all of the opposing views on the news and social media.

Beth was especially confused by the hatred of Chinese people that was visited upon Koreans, Vietnamese, Filipinos, and anyone else who looked even remotely Asian. She understood the zombie poisoning might possibly have come from Chinese food through some infected/contaminated import, but it did not make sense to worry about freshly made Chinese food from local restaurants. After all, there had been many cases of domestic and imported food, like romaine lettuce, contaminated with Listeria, E. coli, or Salmonella and had nothing to do with China. So, it was not entirely out of the realm of possibility that some food imported from China might make people sick. The zombie connection, however, was strange to Beth. She decided to look into this a bit more. The drapes in her bedroom had a vaguely Asian pattern, were bright red, and at night looked like the Chinese dragons one sees at the New Year's festivals. She wondered if that could be dangerous. It was worth pondering. She wondered if she was having a premonition. The pondering felt different than normal, letting her mind wander or concentrating on trying to solve a problem. It was as if her brain was an engine that wouldn't turn over. Her thoughts were taking more effort than usual. She felt and heard a buzzing throughout her brain and body. It was like she was receiving a message.

Beth wondered if she might be psychic. After all, the "Something's Coming" song has been going through her head for months. Maybe she had had a vision. She should go buy a lottery ticket. But, since she didn't have a vision of the winning lottery numbers, she decided to stay home. The outside world was getting strange. Too strange to feel safe. Something was definitely not right, and she wasn't sure what to do.

Even stranger was the unusual number of friend requests she was getting on social media. She didn't know any of the people. While they had different names and locations, they all were unusually thin men, and in every photo, they were wearing some version of a bulky blue sweater. She was looking to make more connections, so she replied in the affirmative to their requests on all social media platforms. Their messages have been so flattering she just can't say no. Over the past month or two, she's become busier and busier chatting online with these men. They make her feel better about herself. They seem kind, and they constantly are telling her how beautiful she is. It's sad none of them live near her. They all seem to work outside of the United States. It's too bad their internet doesn't work well because then she could video chat instead of messaging, but they all complain about their poor internet. So, it must be true. Why would they lie to her?

Thoroughly enjoying her nighttime ritual of social media and chatting with her new friends, Beth decided she should spend more time on social media and probably shouldn't watch TV so close to bedtime. Every night, her dreams were overrun by visions of zombie apocalypses and alien invasions. Her dreams are extremely detailed and vivid. She can't always tell who's a real person and who is a zombie impersonating them. It's frightening. Normally, when she has terrible nightmares, she can turn on the TV and watch something mindless to relax. But now, the channel surfing is inundated with images of death, destruction, and zombies. Strangely enough, the TV shows about aliens living among humanity, while they may start out with the aliens trying to kill the human race, always end up with the aliens being the good guys. It was confusing and exceedingly difficult to tell the difference between the news, reality TV, and scripted TV, and none of it was particularly helpful in getting Beth to relax and fall back asleep.

After watching one too many reality TV shows, at least she thought it was a reality TV show; it may have been the news, Beth decided the reasonable thing to do was to prepare for a zombie apocalypse and build up supplies in her house with a stockpile worthy of the stars of *Extreme Couponers* — an idea she got from late-night television watching. She became obsessed with the idea of building a stockpile. She watched the TV show over and over, analyzing what kinds of products the professional shoppers had in their stockpiles, looking at which stores they shopped, studied how they rotated their stock so she could make her own plans. There were a few technical difficulties she would have to overcome, but Beth wasn't particularly good at figuring out how to completely implement a plan anymore. So the fact she did not subscribe to any newspapers from which to clip coupons didn't bother her, nor did the fact that none of the grocery stores within one hundred miles of her doubled coupons. She obsessed over building a stockpile to protect against zombies.

Beth didn't spend all her time watching TV and preparing for zombies, however. She had spent hours upon hours over the past month chatting with her new Facebook friends. She got messages from them multiple times a day. And after chatting for a month, she decided she liked Jim. He seemed totally fascinating. He was a doctor with an international organization, and although he said he couldn't give her many details about his job because of the types of places he was in, he was interested in everything about her and attentive. Even though he had a busy job as a doctor working internationally, he managed to message her at least a dozen times a day. He was handsome, and he was into dogs. Beth loved dogs. And, of course, she was impressed that he was a doctor who traveled around the world making things better for people. She was curious, however. She had worked in the healthcare industry for years, albeit on the periphery. She knew most of the medical schools in the United States. Jim was evasive about where he went to school, where he did his residency and his specialty. She'd asked those questions, and he would divert her attention by discussing the dogs he'd seen that day. The diversion always worked. It is odd, though. That diversion would never have worked on Beth when she was younger.

She didn't press the issue because she didn't want to seem like she was interrogating Jim. He seemed nice, she didn't have a social life, and he was good-looking. She also didn't press the issue of religion. She only dated Jewish men, and that's who she was looking for in a life partner. She had asked him a few times if he was Jewish, and he answered that he had "a great interest in the Jewish faith." That choice of words is usually a clue to Jewish people that the person they're talking to isn't Jewish. But, again, this was something for Beth to overlook because she liked this guy.

Beth had had such a bizarre month that she decided to enjoy Jim's attention. She had multiple missteps, quite literally, and tripped over her own feet a couple of times. But, the worst part was when she pulled into her garage, misjudged the distance, and banged into the shelving at the front of her car. Fortunately, all she did was bend the front license plate a bit. Nothing on the shelves was seriously damaged because she hit the edge of the shelving unit itself and the 12-pack of paper towels next to it. She could have been in real trouble if she'd hit the shelving with the canned goods on it. She was aggravated with herself for making what she thought was a "boneheaded" mistake. She attributed it to not paying attention. The first time, that is. The second time it happened that month, she thought she should make an eye doctor appointment. But, it slipped her mind, and she never did. There was so much turmoil in the world, and Beth was easily distracted these days, so it was natural that she forgot to be worried about her depth perception/vision. Instead, she was preoccupied with building up her stockpile. She smiled to herself as she thought of the word "stockpile" because that is the word people featured on the TV show *Extreme Couponers* use to describe their hoards. Maybe she had learned something from watching the show, after all.

Out of an abundance of caution, Beth decided to take a rideshare service to the gourmet grocery store. She had everything she needed for the zombie apocalypse, or so she thought. But she honestly was bored with everything she was cooking, and quite unreasonably, she couldn't find anything she wanted to eat from the 276 restaurants that delivered. Hence, the ride to the gourmet grocery store. She used to love their bistro meals where customers could choose from a huge selection of chef-prepared entrées, vegetables, and starches to create their own custom-made meal. The food was delicious, although quite expensive, and the options varied. So, Beth thought this might be worthy of an adventure. About halfway to the store, she realized the same silent, motionless man from the Las Vegas taxi was sitting next to her in the backseat. She thought it was strange because she hadn't ordered a communal car from the rideshare service, but she was already halfway there, so she decided not to worry. It's interesting that her only thought was about the type of rideshare she had ordered, not that there was a strange person sitting next to her. Nor did it even register that it was unusual for her to recognize this man, that he still was silent and motionless, and she was able to recognize the clothing he was wearing as the same as he wore in that short ride in the taxi in Las Vegas. In her defense, however, Beth had other things on her mind. She had forgotten her shopping list. While she knew she would choose the bistro meals from what was available in the prepared food case, she couldn't remember what else she needed. Milk? Fruit? Bread? Trying to reconstruct her shopping list for a gourmet grocery store that didn't carry the usual essentials occupied most of her brain space. There wasn't much room left for the strange man sitting next to her.

4

APRIL - PREPARING FOR THE APOCALYPSE

Beth decided to brave the full-sized grocery store one last time in order to create a stockpile to protect against the impending zombie apocalypse. The preparation was getting a bit obsessive. Worse yet, there was a flaw in her plan. There were multiple flaws. The first was that she had not counted on the grocery store being as stressful, crowded, and complicated as it was the last time she had gone. The second was that she had never clipped coupons in her life, had no idea how to start, and therefore didn't bring any coupons. She would have failed as a guest on *Extreme Couponers*. The resulting shopping trip was extremely expensive and exhausting. But, at the end of the day, she had filled the trunk and backseat of her car with things she thought she might need if she were stuck in her house, avoiding zombies. Or, at least she could be hospitable to the zombies or aliens if they were the "something's coming."

Once again, she found another piece of sea glass in the parking lot. It was exactly the same shape as the other two. She used to be fascinated by sea glass when she was younger, and seeing it reminded her of summers on the beaches of New England. It did strike her as odd that she was nowhere near the ocean but kept finding pieces of sea glass, and the shape of the sea glass was unusual. She was used to finding chunks of sea glass that had been smoothed by the waves, but she had never seen round, flat discs with a concave impression on the top. Yet, she had found three pieces of the same shape recently. She remembered that in her youth, she and her friends would collect shells and sea glass along the beach and keep them in glass jars instead of leaving them loose. So, she stopped at the craft store near the grocery store and picked up a glass jar with a lid for her new treasures. She was so intent on finding a parking space near the craft store that she didn't recognize that once again, after touching the sea glass, her fingers and arm tingled, and it went all the way up to her head, and she became dizzy. The strange sensations persisted the entire time she was in the craft store looking at jars and the whole time she drove home.

Once she returned home, she evaluated her garage. Or, as she called it, her overflow kitchen. It's attached to her regular kitchen and has an extra refrigerator/freezer, a chest freezer, and shelves that host the items that don't fit in her regular kitchen. She was convinced that an extremely tall gremlin who only ate canned food had designed the cabinets in the real kitchen. You need to be six feet tall to reach anything above the second shelf, and the shelves themselves are at odd heights that cannot fit a cereal box, a bag of potato chips, or anything else useful. So, anything nonperishable lives on the shelves in the garage. Anything that didn't fit in her small side-by-side refrigerator/freezer combination in the kitchen lived in the better-designed refrigerator/freezer combo and the chest freezer in the garage. Yes, she lived alone and had three freezers and two refrigerators when one adds up the combinations. In her defense, however, she liked to entertain and did so often.

As she admired her handiwork in organizing her stockpile of food and supplies, she was reminded of that famous scene in *Willy Wonka and the Chocolate Factory* with the chocolate river, the candy mushrooms filled with whipped cream, and the giant lollipops. In her garage, that scene contains giant packages of toilet paper, mountains of paper towels, a truckload of sanitizing wipes, a towering display of 30-gallon garbage bags, buckets of laundry soap and dishwashing soap tablets, and a fantasyland of cleaning products. Mixed in among the candy and the chocolate and the household products, she has what seem like millions of cans of tuna, fruit, pudding, and vegetables. But the crowning glory of it all is the ice cream, cookies, and whipped cream piled high in the freezer with as much of everything as you would want. She certainly wouldn't want to run out of treats during a zombie apocalypse.

The walls are lined with cases of Diet Coke®, which form a maze zigzagging around the apocalypse preparation fantasy world. As she travels this route, she sees the family of toy bears, pink bunnies, and unicorns who live in the corner. They're friendly; she liberated them from the pet store last Christmas. In Beth's defense, they were on sale, and they were a favorite toy of all dogs who came to visit. She had plenty for the dogs to take home with them. She wasn't quite sure where these stuffed animals fit in the scheme of preparing for a zombie apocalypse. In the midst of reviewing her stash, even she had to admit it probably was not relevant. She did buy them for a fundraiser that got canceled. But, they added to the general feel of absurdity.

Depending on your outlook, that general feel of absurdity, hoarding, or preparation was further enhanced by the Christmas tree collection also housed in the garage. Nestled between two big bins of ornaments housed on the round white extra dining room table that lived in the garage were eight 18-inch tabletop Christmas trees guarded by two giant stuffed bears in sweaters. Stacked below the table were a dozen 36-inch Christmas trees in boxes. They were guarded by two particularly interesting gnomes. They looked like a hybrid between a gnome and a Christmas tree. They looked friendly, not appearing like the most menacing guards. The most ridiculous thing of many ridiculous things in this apocalypse preparation fantasy world was the presence of so many Christmas decorations. Beth is Jewish. She doesn't celebrate Christmas. Nor did she ever put up Christmas trees. It was for a fundraiser. But zombie apocalypses and fundraisers don't go hand-in-hand.

While Beth admired her handiwork and preparation, she got a phone call from her parents and sister. They were deeply concerned about Beth and her ability to survive a zombie apocalypse. They clearly didn't think she had enough stuff in her garage, even though she video-called them to show what she had. They were particularly concerned about toilet paper, freezer bags, foaming hand soap, disinfecting wipes, and tuna fish. They were beyond worried, however, about protein shakes and fig bars, Beth's breakfast of choice. And they were right to worry — both about her having protein shakes and fig bars every morning for breakfast and the limited amount she had on hand. Two cases of each would last one month. However, there was positively no way at all Beth was going to attempt to go to Costco or anywhere like that. She learned her lesson at the regular grocery store. She told her parents and sister not to worry, told them she would go online and have everything delivered to her house, and reminded them that they had seen everything she had stored in her garage. If it was enough to make her think of a scene from *Willy Wonka*, it was enough to supply her for a while. At least, that's what she thought...

Finally admitting they were right to worry, Beth searched high and low for protein shakes and fig bars. It was impossible to get any of the things they worried about. Beth had to call for help and have her sister find them. It took more than a month to get everything she needed. For some reason, the whole world panicked about toilet paper and Diet Coke®. True confession... In two weeks, Beth had eaten all of the sugar-free Jell-O® from her stockpile. Now, she stared sadly at the empty display case. She couldn't find any more to refill it. It appeared that even a year later, there still were shortages, and that included gelatin.

The one positive thing was her blossoming relationship with Jim. If his internet connection were better, she'd be much happier. She would like to video chat with him at some point. But his sweet messages, which he sent her multiple times a day, always put a smile on her face. Beth thought she might be falling in love. He was so thoughtful. For example, she'd wake up in the morning to a message that says, "Good morning, my love." When she would message back, he would inevitably respond with, "Did you dream of me, my love? I dreamed of you!" He finally gave Beth more information about himself. He said he was an orthopedic surgeon working for the United Nations in Syria, and a widower with a young daughter who was with him. Beth's heart went out to him. Clearly, he was a good guy trying to raise a kid alone in Syria and working as an orthopedic surgeon. She started spending more and more time texting him. He always seemed to respond, even with the seven-hour time difference. She wondered when he slept. But, she was thrilled he took the time to talk with her — always.

It was a strange time of year for Beth. She was used to hosting Passover Seders* and had for decades. She usually hosted at least 20-25 people a night for the two traditional Seders, and often hosted an additional twenty for leftovers on the third night. She enjoyed sharing the tradition of enjoying special foods, drinking wine, telling stories and even singing a few traditional songs.

This year, the fear of zombies kept people at home. She made a modified dinner for herself. She had done a lot of the grocery shopping in February when she thought she still would be hosting Passover. The 22-pound turkey was sitting in the bottom of her freezer. The five-pound package of matzoh was sitting on a shelf in her garage while the twenty pounds of assorted matzoh cooking products were sitting nearby, surrounding the ten jars of Kosher for Passover jam that was supposed to be turned into a jellyroll. The chicken for the chicken soup was sitting in the second, smaller freezer. And, she had no one to eat it with her. She was glad she had never made it to the kosher supermarket or to Costco to get the rest of the items because clearly anything perishable was going to perish. She couldn't possibly eat twenty pounds of potatoes or onions. It wasn't worth making an entire vat of chicken soup and matzoh balls, so she skipped that as well.

As she sat alone at the table, eating dinner, she decided she needed to take out one Seder plate. Traditionally, there may be one plate or several. The procedure is detailed in a book called a *Haggadah*, which may be written in Hebrew, Arabic, or even English. Following tradition, she chose one set of candlesticks and her Elijah's cup. She often shared with new guests the story of Elijah who was traditionally seen as the herald of the messianic age, which originates from a second-century debate among the sages over whether there should be four or five cups of wine, based on the number of promises between God and the enslaved Israelites. To address this uncertainty, the *Haggadah* introduced "the cup of Elijah" as a symbolic fifth cup. Besides his expected role in announcing the messianic age, Elijah is revered in Jewish folklore as a miraculous savior and intercessor for the Jewish people, making his presence symbolically important at various Jewish ceremonies, especially the Passover Seder. It didn't seem like a holiday at all, otherwise.

The tradition at Beth's Seders had been to pour wine into the Elijah's cup. Then, during the Seder, the children would open the front door to let Elijah in. While the children were distracted looking out the door, one of the adults would drink the wine from the Elijah's cup. When the children returned to the table, disappointed they hadn't seen Elijah, the adults would point out that clearly, he had snuck past them because he had finished the wine from his cup.

Beth's family took that tradition one step further. At least fifty years ago, Beth's grandmother was roasting chickens for Passover. Her reputation had been that she overcooked everything. Legend has it that her rule of thumb was "cook it until it's done, and then cook it for another hour." That rule was hard and fast for any meat or poultry.

At Passover, she also had to juggle the timing of when the food was done versus when the men had finished reading the entire *Haggadah*. It took hours. And the whole time, the chickens were roasting away in the oven. Naturally, the chickens burned. And as could be expected when the chickens are burning in the oven, smoke poured out of the oven. Fortunately, Beth's grandmother had left the window near the oven open so the house did not completely fill up with smoke. The Seder continued as if nothing was wrong until the children opened the door for Elijah, that is.

Once, standing in the doorway was a firefighter, in full gear. He and the rest of his team had seen smoke pouring out the window. They decided to see if everything was okay. Since then, the story is retold every year at Passover in every home of Beth's grandmother's relatives. The story has survived from generation to generation.

This year, in keeping with tradition, even though she was alone, Beth set out Elijah's cup and opened the door looking for him, or the fire department. She was convinced this time Elijah was going to be there. Nothing would have been able to convince her otherwise. Leaving the door open the entire time she was having dinner, she had a full conversation with Elijah, even going so far as to take out a second plate and place setting in case he was hungry. She was sure he had sipped some of the wine because she knew there was less in the cup than she had put there originally. And she was comforted.

It was as if her brain was split in two. Part was convinced Elijah was having dinner with her, and the other part was trying to break through, pointing out that this was absurd. Beth thought to herself:

The buzzing is back. It's the craziest thing. I feel a buzzing in my brain, and I get this overwhelming sense of déjà vu. Feeling, not sound. It's like a memory I can't quite place my finger on. I feel it more than I know it — like that gut instinct we have that something's not quite right and the hair on the back of our neck stands up. It also seems like what we used to call a "snowy picture" on TV. You could kind of see the picture behind the snow, and could kind of hear the audio, but it wasn't at all clear. My brain feels like that when it buzzes.

So, my brain is buzzing again. This time I can at least figure out the reason — it's the man sitting next to me. I KNOW that I know him from somewhere. Can't place him. He seems so familiar. I feel like I should know him, but I don't. The feeling of déjà vu is overwhelming, but the memory itself is out of reach.

But, then I look into his eyes. He's staring earnestly into my eyes like he's trying to send me a message. It's strange. I feel like I've known him forever. The buzzing in my brain is on overload. Who the hell is this man? Why do I feel like I know him when I don't?

But, I want to know him. I want to know who this man is, sitting by my side, holding my hand. He's clearly trying to take care of me. He's offering me something to drink, but I'm not thirsty. He offers me some food, but I'm not hungry. I feel safe with him here. I somehow know he'll protect me.

I don't know who he is, but I don't want to see the sadness in his eyes. Why is he so sad when he looks at me? I want to see him happy. I don't understand why I care. I have no idea who this stranger is, but he seems kind. This whole time, he's only said one thing to me: "It's not quite time yet." I have no idea what he means, but for some strange reason, I'm disappointed.

As he leaves, I see him put a handful of sea glass in the Elijah's cup. It's beautiful. What a thoughtful gift.

5

MAY - SPRINGTIME DURING THE APOCALYPSE

    It's early springtime in Washington, D.C. That means three important things: the weather is entirely unpredictable and can have 40° temperature swings, the cherry blossoms come out and viewing them is a huge social event, and the pollen count spikes to create an entirely miserable experience for any of us who have allergies or asthma. Many people wear masks outside to protect themselves from the pollen, as they have done for years.

    Normally, Beth was careful about going outside when the pollen turned her car green. But she had moved to a new neighborhood with wonderful sidewalks, great neighbors, and new areas to explore. So, she took her chances. It wasn't a wise move, but it was beautiful. It was fitting that it was springtime. Beth's thoughts flit like butterflies throughout her mind. They're impossible to catch and hold on to, although she can see them, sense them, and feel them. But they won't stay still for a second. She can't hang on to her thoughts like she can't catch the butterflies she sees fluttering around her.

The neighborhood has a certain etiquette — the dogs are great social connectors. For example, if you are home and want visitors, you leave your garage door open, and the dogs will walk right in. Or, they will bark at your front door to see if you are home. When you are on a walk, they greet every single person they see. Even though Beth doesn't have a dog, she does have dog treats and toys in her house for any canine visitors. Embarking on a walk involves preparation: making sure to grab the cell phone and that it's charged, dressing appropriately to see neighbors, and putting a baggie full of dog cookies in the fanny pack. Of course, since it's open season for pollen, a mask and sunglasses also are a necessity. One wouldn't want to be caught unprepared, and the dogs do check everyone they pass to see if that person has treats.

It may seem unusual for anyone to worry about what they wear (dressing appropriately) when walking in their own neighborhood. Once upon a time, Beth didn't care. Then she learned her lesson. Earlier this year, she had spent a long day on conference calls and at the computer. It was a beautiful day at the end of January and much warmer than could be expected. She had been working from home, wasn't showered, in dirty, ill-fitting sweatpants and a stained sweatshirt. Her hair was uncombed, and she shouldn't have been seen in public like that. This was one of those put-your-lipstick-on-before-you-go-check-your-mail neighborhoods, after all. But, she was going to take a quick walk around the block and didn't want to miss the end of daylight by taking the time to change her clothes and do her hair. She figured no one would see her at that time of day. So she left the house dressed like a slob and looking like she had had a rough night out.

Of course, she was wrong about not seeing any neighbors. Very wrong. Murphy's Law was alive and well that day. She ran into four neighbors who were impeccably dressed and on their way to a concert when they stopped to chat with her. Then, when she was on her way home, a fire truck and ambulance came up behind her. She quickly stepped out of the middle of the street where she had been walking and into her driveway to allow them to pass. Much to her surprise, they stopped in her cul-de-sac. Then, the EMTs and firefighters came out.

As did six of Beth's neighbors who came rushing out to make sure she was okay since the ambulance and fire truck had stopped in front of her house. Beth couldn't figure out why the fire trucks and ambulances were there. Perhaps she had dropped her emergency pendant she had partially set up after thinking it was a good idea to purchase since she lived alone — and losing interest in completing the process? Hit the emergency call button on her cell phone while walking?

The answer had nothing to do with anything like that. Instead, there were new ambulance and fire truck drivers and they were practicing driving down small streets and making U-turns in the cul-de-sac without hitting the fire hydrant. Her driveway apparently is exactly the right spot to aim the nose of the truck to avoid hitting the fire hydrant. While the driver was maneuvering, the rest of the teams in the ambulance and fire truck were standing in the street and in Beth's driveway, directing the driver. Beth learned her lesson that day and swore she would never walk out of the house dressed like that again. Not only did all of her neighbors see her dressed and unkempt, but so did the entire fire battalion. Beth had to call her mother and admit she was right. She always said, "Don't go out of the house without combing your hair!"

That day, however, Beth made sure she was dressed appropriately, had dog cookies and her phone, and decided to see exactly how far she could walk. She headed out through her quiet neighborhood and walked along the sidewalk. Two neighbors were out in their yards pulling weeds. Another was wiping off the benches in the little park where the flowers were beginning to poke through the mulch. Other neighbors were walking in groups of four or five down the middle of the street — traffic usually is light around here, so it wasn't a problem. Everyone would stop and talk with each other. It was friendly, collegial, and clearly a neighborhood where people knew each other and socialized. The dogs would go up to everybody and see how many dog treats they could get. One dog preferred to be at home, and after she scored as many treats as she could, would take her leash and leave. She never ran away. She would take her leash and go home. But otherwise, most of the dogs were happy to stand around and socialize with each other and the humans.

After walking out of the neighborhood, Beth carefully crossed over the main street. Doing so always is frightening. There is a stop sign, but no traffic light, and many of the drivers zoom through without using signals. Beth's house is on that corner, and she hears car crashes on a regular basis. She always is relieved when they hit each other instead of the tree in front of her house, or the signs on the median strip. While the tree poses an obvious danger of falling on her house if it's hit, the danger of hitting the signs is less obvious. Inevitably, the signs go flying across the street and usually hit another car and get dangerously close to hitting pedestrians if they aren't fast enough to get out of the way. Beth has had some near misses on that corner.

On this particular day, the ornamental pear trees were stunning. The trees are at least twenty-five years old, line both sides of the street, and form a tunnel/canopy of beautiful white flowers. It's this neighborhood's version of the cherry blossoms that grace other streets and neighborhoods in the D.C. area. Beth was happily enjoying her walk, enjoying her neighbors, and in general, appreciating the day. In contrast to the glory of the pear trees, the forsythia, and the daffodils, Beth's yard didn't look so good. In her defense, when she first moved in, she had paid someone to pull up dead bushes, prune things that clearly hadn't been touched in decades, and clean up the yard. However, she had wanted to see if any perennials would bloom in the spring before she dug things up. She recognized that her yard looked as bad as her outfit did when the fire trucks came. It was going to take a lot of work to clean up this mess. It seemed strange to be worrying about the yard in the context of zombie apocalypse preparation, which still was on every news channel. However, it was so beautiful outside that it was easy to forget about the zombies or whatever form the predicted apocalypse was going to take. The yard work, however, was immediately obvious.

These were the days before the predicted zombie apocalypse was clearly understood. It was a time when humanity got away with a little preparation, limiting exposure in large crowds, and not much else. So, today's walk was a walk like any other day. Beth and her neighbors were discussing transplanting azaleas and rhododendrons, deciding how many more lavender plants Beth needed, and wondering if the rosebushes would come back. The other topics of conversation involved whether the deer were going to eat everything in sight, whether the squirrels ate the hostas or if the deer could be blamed, and if any houses were going to be on the market soon. It seemed Beth was finding more and more sea glass in unusual locations, particularly on these walks. She always gathered it, and her jar was filling up. She would take off the lid and fidget with the pieces of sea glass as if they were worry stones. In the beginning, it would calm her. Then, the tingling and headaches would start. Beth never made the connection.

This day and this walk would be repeated over and over again. The topics would change as the wildlife emerged from their hibernation and began eating the lawns and landscaping. One day the conversation was hostas, the second day it was daffodils, and the third day it was admiring the chutzpah of the deer that literally congregated in a group watching the humans. The deer contentedly ate every newly budding plant in one of the yards while the humans stared in amazement. But in general, it was all benign, neighborly conversations — standard social interactions and checking in with each other. By the way, the only plants that seemed to remain completely untouched by both deer and squirrels were the horseradish.

Beth had a flashback to a close friend of hers who was on a personal mission to get revenge on the deer who had eaten her eighteen rosebushes in less than thirty minutes. That friend had a habit of running out of her house with her hair in curlers, wearing a housecoat and slippers, and banging on a pot with a wooden spoon while screaming at the deer every time she saw them. Standing with her neighbors, watching the deer destroy thousands of dollars in landscaping, Beth was torn between understanding her friend's reaction and enjoying the deer. Her neighbors seemed to tend toward enjoying the deer.

The neighbors continued their conversation and made plans for happy hour in the neighborhood park, pizza in the park, times to walk together on different routes, plans to go to new restaurants, and vague mentions of hoping the zombie apocalypse had been prevented. Most people were happy the weather was nice and they could come out of winter hibernation.

Beth's neighborhood, in general, was more aware of the impending apocalypse and what it could do since it was an over-fifty community, and some neighbors are well into their nineties. But, it was more of a watch-and-wait situation instead of panic. In fact, some of the neighbors were looking forward to dead people returning to life and walking among the living. They were old enough they had lost many loved ones, and while a zombie apocalypse could be frightening, it wasn't always that way. Besides, everyone had enough toilet paper. People had so many supplies they traded them among neighbors.

And, when the new neighbors moved in, everyone offered to share supplies with them, as well. There were at least three new families who moved in during this period. They were rather nondescript. When the usual walking group got together to gossip, in a truly kind manner, about the new neighbors, they were difficult to describe. "Bland," if one were to have to choose one word. There were three couples; all of whom were tall and thin, and they all shared a fondness for bulky blue sweaters and jeans. No one was being judgmental; they were stating facts. It was common for someone to say, "I like your hair," "Is that a new winter coat?" or "Did you get a new car?" It was a matter of conversation. People watched out for each other in this neighborhood, and they noticed things.

Walks and conversations over the next few weeks were relatively similar, and then Beth found the squirrel family. They clearly were having a reunion. It was in her front yard. They were happily devouring all ninety-eight of her newly planted petunias. They had carefully dug them up from the ground and placed them in a big pile to make them easier to eat. Then, they tried to come in the screen door in the sunroom. Apparently, they wanted something else to eat to complement the petunias. Perhaps they saw the Amazon delivery of the trail mix and wanted some.

The squirrel family was friendly. They always welcomed her and chattered away when she walked by a family gathering. They also made a point of sitting outside the sliding glass door in her sunroom and chattering at her. On the days when the screen door was closed but the glass was open, they would put their little fingers on the screen and try to open it. Clearly, they were used to hanging out in her house. Perhaps that had been when the previous owner was there because she doesn't remember ever inviting them. But, she enjoyed her conversations with them. Recently, though, their chatter has been more and more agitated, and they've been manic about storing nuts and seeds and popcorn and going through the trash. It was odd behavior for this time of year. Beth wondered if they knew what the big thing was that was coming… Is it possible the signs were only visible to squirrels?

She was mildly surprised when she saw two squirrels dragging an entire box of cereal down the street. Beth heard a tremendous amount of clanking, banging, chattering, and footsteps on the roof of her sunroom, and then she swore she heard the same in her attic. Her assumption was that she had tenants. Tenants of the squirrel kind, that is. That was a turning point for Beth. And apparently, it was a turning point for the squirrels, as well. They weren't just squirrels; they were roommates who became Beth's friends. They'd accompany her on walks, chattering away all the while. They would sit on the lawn next to the driveway when Beth had been out doing errands and wait for her return. She bought extra food she thought they'd like and left it outside in her yard near the trellis they used to climb up to the attic. They still had difficulty distinguishing between the weeds Beth wanted them to eat and the flowers she wished they wouldn't, but in general the friendship was working out.

Suddenly, the music in Beth's head stopped. She hadn't realized exactly how persistent the *West Side Story* music had been until it ended. At first, she was shocked by the unrelenting silence. For months, the music accompanied her wherever she went. While in the beginning, she had thought of it as something fun and romantic and happily anticipated the something that was coming, most recently she had found it disturbing and frightening. She was afraid of what was coming. She was right.

It's difficult to believe so much has happened in such a short amount of time. Beth's world, indeed, most of planet Earth, has changed drastically since March. The 24-hour news cycle repeatedly commented on how decimated the greater New York City area has been. The zombies clearly have gone on the attack. People were given varied, often contradictory, information about how to protect themselves from being turned into zombies and what type of equipment they needed to remain safe. The panic created by this confusing information was further exacerbated by the utter lack of protective equipment. It was a real-life "Chicken Little" situation; the sky was falling, but the commentators had been inciting panic for months, so no one knew what to believe. And the zombies laughed as the humans were driven into panic. The humans were so busy panicking they missed opportunities to stop the zombie apocalypse, defied logic, and pandered to the panic.

Some people, and some industries, however, took prudent action based on what they knew about zombies or other contagions such as viruses, bacterial infections, etc. Nursing homes, assisted living communities, and senior housing/retirement communities, for example, instituted no-visitor policies and that struck home for many of Beth's friends and neighbors who have loved ones in those communities. They didn't think it was fair that they couldn't visit. And, they worried about their loved ones being scared or lonely.

On the other hand, Beth and many of her healthcare provider friends were grateful some people were being prudent. Traditionally, zombies infect other people in ways similar to Leprosy, Legionnaires' disease, and bioterrorism. Beth's friends understood how viruses and bacterial infections spread, and at that point, conventional wisdom said people who lived in communities of older adults were less likely to effectively fight off zombies than were young healthy people. So, it made sense to treat a zombie apocalypse like an infection and to implement strict infection control procedures, the same way one would if there were a measles or smallpox outbreak.

Scientists, still unsure about exactly which techniques the zombies were using, decided treating the zombie apocalypse as if it were a virus made sense. The lockdowns were the result of logistics. Considering how many types of people go in and out of these communities, it was easy to see how they could be zombie converters/carriers and infect multiple communities. This led to many philosophical discussions about the undead, the recently departed, the soon to be departing, and the relationship among them. Not everyone was convinced the zombies were bad.

There was significant debate about whether the world was at the beginning of a zombie apocalypse or an alien invasion or both. Was this the beginning of times? Was this the end of times? There were debates among religious leaders of all sects around the world.

Conventional wisdom said the zombies had to touch someone in order for that person to be converted. The general rule of thumb, according to the pundits, was to stay six feet away from other people, in case they are zombies and want to convert you. Of course, any self-respecting zombie will tell you that they don't infect you by coughing on you. They don't need to get that close. They are much better, efficient, and effective at recruiting new zombies than they're given credit for. And, in no zombie movie ever do the zombies take over the world person by person, one person at a time.

In Beth's world, however, many people are lemmings and often don't pay attention or think for themselves. People could not differentiate between real zombie protocol, hogwash, and fear mongering. So, rather than following logic and reason, many people picked and chose what they felt like doing to protect themselves from the zombies. It seemed as though the more ridiculous the option, the more the lemmings followed it. Many people debated whether the zombies were real even though the hospitals were full of dying zombies, the morgues were full, and in major cities, refrigerated trucks were used to store the bodies of dead zombies. But, as always, determining whether something is real, a delusion, dementia, or a flat-out lie is beyond many people's ability.

And the zombies laughed as grocery stores put tape on the floors to delineate six-foot spacing, limiting the number of people who can go into the store at any one time, and creating one-way aisles to try to space out the shoppers. The zombies found it quite amusing how many people could not follow a directional arrow on the floor or read a sign, no matter what language it was in or what language they spoke. Social gatherings were pretty much eliminated. People were not supposed to visit each other's homes, children were not supposed to have play dates, and in general, people were supposed to self-quarantine.

Many healthcare professionals and political leaders advised people to stay at home unless they needed to go somewhere for something essential. They were trying to avoid having people gather inside, or even outside when social distancing wasn't possible. "Social distancing" was a new term to describe staying six feet away from other people. Somehow or another, the way a virus spreads were hijacked and applied to a zombie apocalypse in addition to the way a social media post spreads, "going viral."

Again, the zombies laughed. They found it particularly amusing that anyone thought the zombies converted people within six feet of them and even funnier that most humans had no idea how far six feet was. They also found it funny what people considered necessary. As in, people were supposed to self-isolate unless going out for something necessary. The zombies, who were monitoring social media, the news, and conversations among people who were gathering, found the entire concept totally hysterical. They did not care why you were outside; they were looking to convert people to zombies. It did not matter if the person was going to church, going to the grocery store for the seventh time that week, or had run out of snack food. They were going to "get you" anyway. The zombies were making bets on how ridiculous the human behavior would get. The people did not let them down with the extent of their ridiculousness.

Humanity was so distracted by the stay-at-home orders and social distancing they didn't pay attention to the sudden influx of silver RVs floating along the highways. Even worse, the meteorologists never reported any of the freezing fog becoming more prevalent around the world. Instead, the debate continued about whether the zombies were here, whether the hospitals were full, if one needed to go to the hospital if one came in contact with a zombie, and whether or not someone's "need" to get snacks at the local bodega was an emergency, a God-given right, selfish, life-threatening, or a combination of the above.

The world was teetering on the brink. The brink of what, no one knew. Yet, Beth was happy. Her jar full of sea glass worry stones looked gorgeous in the sunlight. She was finding so much of it that she had to order a larger jar online. She was beginning to think she'd have enough to create a lamp base like they used to fill with seashells on Cape Cod during summers in Massachusetts. This one would be filled with colored sea glass. She was surprised she even had found some of the rarer colors, like dark blue and red. It kept her entertained.

Then, just like that, with no warning, the world became faceless. Beth was comforted by that. Recently, she'd been having trouble recognizing people. It was embarrassing. But, now everyone was told to wear a mask to protect them from the zombies, thus rendering them faceless so it wasn't as obvious that she couldn't remember or recognize people.

She knew it was not particularly risky to take a walk outside, wear a mask, and to go at dusk when everybody else is having dinner so she'd reduce her chances of running into anybody. But today, she couldn't stand sitting at her desk anymore and went for a walk at three o'clock in the afternoon. It was a beautiful, sunny day. She thought the weather was perfect and was happily traipsing around in leggings and a lightweight top. She ran into many of her neighbors. They were bundled up like it was Boston in February. She smiled to herself, completely invisible under her mask, and thought she would have had heatstroke if she dressed that way. Being mindful of social distancing, she stayed six feet away when she talked to them. And she was feeling quite proud of herself because she avoided teasing them about how bundled up they were. She was happy to see most of them were wearing masks. Honestly, though, she suspected they would have been wearing scarves to keep their faces warm if they hadn't been wearing masks. It wasn't necessarily zombie related.

She didn't recognize that some of them, in fact, truly were faceless. All she could see were masks, sunglasses, and hats. Had she taken a closer look, or had they taken off their sunglasses or masks, she would have seen they were faceless. The faceless people looked like aliens. She wasn't sure if she should be worried that aliens appeared to have arrived in her neighborhood. She wasn't even sure they were aliens. Now to wait for the zombies.

Having come across the regular walkers, the usual dogs, and nothing out of the ordinary except the winter-like clothing and facemasks, Beth decided to take a different route than usual. As she turned the corner, she thought she heard music, but it was distant like it was a car radio. She was partially correct. There was a congregation of golf carts in the street. The men sitting in them all had beverages, and one of them had a radio. They each were in their own carts, facing each other with the carts in a circle, each of them had their golf clubs on the back of their carts, and they were just hanging out. The golf course was closed, but they still got together. The difference was they were in the street instead of on the course. Even though the zombies had taken over and had forced the closure of the golf course, and they couldn't go golfing, they found a different solution. Apparently, the actual golfing part of golfing was incidental. Hanging out in the golf carts with a beer or a cocktail apparently was the important part. It gives new meaning to "please don't drink and drive," doesn't it?

Still smiling from the no-golf-involved golf cart gathering, Beth continued her walk and crossed over into the next neighborhood. That neighborhood has extra-wide driveways, wide enough for a 2½-car garage — otherwise known as two cars and a golf cart garage. The first driveway she came to had three golf carts in it with people hanging out. Apparently, it was a different clique than the golf cart circle she had passed earlier. Two driveways over, there was a cocktail party. There were four lawn chairs each six feet apart, TV tray tables, hors d'oeuvres and wine. Each person had their own set-up. They called out to Beth, and she stood on the sidewalk and chatted with them for a while. They had continued their normal socializing but outside and six feet apart. That way no one contaminated anyone else, and everyone's house remained at the same level of cleanliness as it had been. No one had to vacuum, straighten up, or do dishes. This became a ritual in May; they continued to do this every single day at 3:30 p.m. while the weather permitted. Usually, in the past, they had played cards, mah-jongg, or something like that in each other's houses or at the clubhouse, but they hung out and chatted. The female version of the men's "golfing."

The next day, Beth went out to see if the neighborhood she had been in was an aberration. After all, they are single-family homes, the homeowners' association is excellent at creating social events, and therefore, the neighbors know each other. She wanted to see if things were different in the high-rise buildings nearby. Coming out of the neighborhood, Beth took a left instead of a right. She walked along the main street, and this day, there were few cars. People were walking on the sidewalks, on the lawn, and in the street. There were many more people out on that street than in her quiet neighborhood. But people were doing their best to practice social distancing. People who lived in the same house walked together, but the rest of the people were at least a few feet apart.

She had been curious about people in high-rises and how they self-isolated. On a good day, elevators are gross. People touch the buttons, they didn't wash their hands thoroughly after using the bathroom, and now they coughed or touched their face and then touched the buttons. Lobbies are gross as well. The 300 residents who live in those high-rises go in and out of the lobby on a regular basis. Many of them also sit on the chairs, touch the mailboxes, etc. while walking past these buildings,

Beth had to admit to a bit of snarkiness, however. She had heard rumors that some of the homeowners' associations in the high-rises have made rules that dogs cannot walk through the lobby even if they live there. The snarky part of her found it funny that the dogs are regulated when it's the humans who transmit the zombie infestation, not the dogs. So, of course, there was no way Beth was going into the high-rise, but she walked through their parking lots and toward their park. Beth saw no one in the parking lot, no one in the park, and as a matter of fact, no one walking on their side of the street at all. It was weird. Beth puzzled over the reason. She suspected since the people in the high-rises tend to be significantly older, they probably are taking the elevator directly down to their cars in the garage and leaving the building or staying in place entirely. They certainly were not outside being as "social-yet-distanced" as Beth's neighborhood.

Seeing the difference in the two neighborhoods piqued Beth's curiosity. She decided to go exploring. She had tried walking in different directions, and it was interesting, but for some reason, recently, she couldn't walk far enough to see the more distant neighborhoods. Over the past few months, she noticed her right leg was getting more difficult to pick up off the ground. She felt like it was dragging. Some of her neighbors had described something similar and called it "drop-foot." She had been working far too hard to take the time off to go to a doctor. With everything she saw in the news about the zombie infestation spreading, she didn't want to risk going to a doctor. How would she know if the doctor was a zombie, the patients were zombies, or the employees were zombies? It wasn't as if they'd wear a sign saying, "Beware! I'm a zombie..." So, she got in her car to take a drive instead of a walk. Her car is parked in her private garage and is directly attached to her house. She was able to go directly into it, drive around, and then go back directly into her garage without being exposed to anyone or anything. She never left her gated community.

Yes, she recognized that's a totally ridiculous statement. It's not like the zombie infestation is going to get stopped by the gate guard. The thought put a smile on her face. She pictured the poor security guard stopping each car and asking the driver if he was a zombie, a figment of someone's imagination, a criminal, or a resident of her community. Still grinning at the thought, she drove to the other side of the community. She found that people who were in single-family houses were gathered in their parks on lawn chairs six feet apart and socializing. There were many groups of golf carts throughout the community. People in the garden-style apartments were enjoying their gardening. She never saw anybody outside the high-rises.

As she got home, Beth realized she hadn't recognized anyone on her travels. That was strange because she knew a lot of people. Yet, everyone she saw seemed completely nondescript. They didn't have any identifying characteristics or facial features. Normally, she would be fascinated by the types of beards or mustaches, the different shades of lipstick, or the hairstyles she saw on people throughout the day. She brushed the facelessness and nondescriptness off as strange, but figured she was tired and not paying attention.

The next day, Beth decided to explore farther. Later, she recognized how stupid it was. But, the stay-at-home orders specifically said people could go out to do takeout food, drive-through restaurants, grocery shopping, and other essentials. There was positively no way Beth was going into a store for anything. She had learned her lesson after that scary and totally exhausting experience earlier in the year. But the $2 Dunkin' Donuts happy hour specials and their relentless TV commercials made her crave an iced latte. Did she have everything she needed to make her own iced coffee at home? Yes. Would she normally drive to a Dunkin'? No. But she grew up in Boston where Dunkin' Donuts originated, and sometimes she got a craving. So, even though this particular craving was obviously fueled by relentless TV commercials, she thought to herself, "Why not go out for a completely ridiculous reason? Go through the Dunkin' drive-through!" So, she did. They were wearing masks and gloves. She handed them exact change because she didn't want them touching her credit card after they touched somebody else's.

She later found out that for the entire months of March and April, Dunkin' was giving out free doughnuts with the purchase of a beverage. She didn't need to know that. Beth's state, per the governor's orders, was at the point that the police were stopping people to make sure they were going out for essential reasons. Beth was sure she would die of embarrassment admitting to the police that she thought coffee and a doughnut was an essential reason. "Seriously, no one can make the argument that a doughnut is essential, necessary, or anything else like that," she thought to herself. "There might be a case for coffee, however." Later, she smiled at how wrong she was. There was a persistent stereotype that police officers liked to hang out in places that served coffee and donuts when they were off duty. While it's not true, it still could have been an amusing reason for Beth to be out, she mused.

Beth realized she had given far too much attention and energy to the doughnut debate. She recognized there were other things she should be worrying about. It seemed as though the zombies had united and they had planned a coordinated attack. The zombies were getting more efficient and effective as time went on, and their conversion rate was growing exponentially. In most countries throughout the world, people were told to stay at home unless it positively was necessary to go out. It was silly when you think of it. Did the zombies care why the person was outside of their home? Did they stop and say to themselves, "This person must be going out for an essential reason, so let's leave him or her alone?" Or, were the zombies grateful their job was made easier? And, because a person was in their own home didn't make them safe. Or did it?

There weren't any real answers. The scientists were busily researching, the politicians were busily debating and making policy, the defense industry was busily ramping up, the self-proclaimed "experts" who had no expertise but were proliferating social media were hawking their wares, and they all had different policies, procedures, goals, and tactics. They often conflicted. Humanity was arguing among itself about who was right, who was wrong, who was lying, were there miracle cures, did we need miracle cures, etc. And, once again, the zombies laughed. Humanity's lack of a coordinated response to the zombie apocalypse entertained the zombies to no end. They thought it was even funnier than the man-made zombie movies they watched with much glee.

Coffee and doughnut craving notwithstanding, Beth was incredibly careful not to go anywhere since the stay-at-home order was instituted and took extremely limited excursions for the month prior. Beth was fond of telling anyone who would listen that she was more afraid of other people than she was of zombies, alien abduction, being hit by a meteor, or being eaten by a recently defrosted dinosaur. People's responses to crises always had amazed her. She was fond of telling anyone who would listen, "One should never underestimate the moron factor of the human race." She always had been fascinated by people who needed to be told to wash their hands, to cover their noses and mouths if they cough or sneeze, not to pick their noses in public, and not to cough on other people. She was ecstatic the day she learned a new term: "Zombidiot." That one word explains it all and sounds much cooler than "moron factor." She felt vindicated in her snarkiness because there were so many people who behaved so stupidly that the urban dictionary coined this new term to describe people who needed to be taught basic polite human social interaction 101; and the term, like most urban dictionary terms, "went viral."

Beth found it particularly funny that the word "viral" is positive in the social media context and negative in the spread of disease context. She was dismayed, rather than amused, however, at how many people did not understand the term "going viral" was based on the behavior of a virus which spreads person-to-person and in real life, "going viral" is a bad thing. No matter how she simplified it, and she had gotten down to the basics, she could not get some people to understand that while getting more followers to like and share a social media post, i.e., "going viral" was good in the social media world, the spread of measles, polio, and smallpox, i.e., "viral spread" in the real world was bad.

On a similar note, she was equally as dismayed by how many people were too young to remember the old shampoo commercial which explained how people learned about the shampoo: "She told two friends, and they told two friends, and they told two friends, and so on, and so on, and so on." It was accompanied by pictures of a woman holding the shampoo bottle. The number of pictures on the screen grew exponentially until the screen was filled. Beth obsessed for weeks trying to remember what shampoo commercial she was recalling. She knew it was somewhere in the back of her mind, but she could not remember which shampoo it was.

She frantically searched online and never found the answer. But, along the way, she went down the rabbit hole of social media and internet searches. She spent hours with one search leading to another which led to yet another, and so on and so on, and so on. Just like the commercial. The information overload totally overwhelmed her. After a while, she forgot what she was looking for, and couldn't keep track of whether she was on a legitimate news site, a fiction or fantasy site, or reading a blog of someone's delusional thinking.

Fantasy, reality, delusions, political and/or religious zeal, fiction, truth, and sheer idiocy became indistinguishable. As Beth dove deeper into the rabbit hole, she saw things on the internet she thought were unbelievable. They were too stupid to be real. But, many people are so ridiculous that they post their antics on social media in the hopes they and their posts can "go viral" in the social media sense, because they think that's important. And other people believe them.

Examples include: the lick-the-toilet challenge to "prove" that viral spread/germ spreading in the real world is fake news; the licking door handles to grocery stores videos; as a protest when young people try to get in to stores during the times that were set aside for elderly and those with special needs; people purposely coughing on produce or other items in grocery stores; spring break partiers in Florida; pastors holding church services with more than 500 people in the same room even after they were warned the zombies had already infiltrated; people hosting bonfires with sixty of their "closest" friends to prove that no zombie was going to stop them from doing what they wanted, and when stopped by police and given a warning, the bonfire hosts invited everybody back a second time; and other ridiculous antics. All of this at the same time as the zombies stood by these people and converted them. It was easy pickings, the zombies thought. Some of them were a bit bored by the lack of a challenge. The zombies started appropriating a human expression: "It's like shooting fish in a barrel." "Darwin must be rolling over in his grave," Beth mused. Or, she corrected, "He's probably dancing around saying, 'I told you so! I told you so! I told you so!'" Beth wanted to wear a sweatshirt that says "Darwin" near the Zombidiots. But they wouldn't get it, so she decided not to waste her money.

Beth's obsession with shampoo, the moron factor, and toilet-licking kept her busy. It was interesting that she could concentrate for so many hours while obsessing over these things, yet she didn't manage to settle down long enough to write a single column in two weeks. Instead, her obsession morphed into everything zombie related.

It was clear to Beth the zombies were real and were in her neighborhood. Sometimes, out of the corner of her eye when she's sitting at her desk and working on the computer, she swears she sees a zombie looking in the sunroom window. But with everything she's seeing on the news, the real world seems so bizarre that a zombie peeking in through her sunroom doesn't seem unexpected. Even with that said, though, she can't shake the feeling that something is not quite right. She sees signs that something's not right, signals she thinks are proof the zombies are trying to communicate with her. She most certainly does not want to be mistaken for a conspiracy theorist. The conspiracy theorists are coming out of the woodwork. They've tried to blame the spread of the zombie apocalypse on everything from other people, to food, to governments, to aliens, to meteors, to defrosted dinosaurs from the polar ice caps, to artificial intelligence, to robots, and never to human behavior or the zombies themselves. So, while Beth thinks something is not quite right with her and her surroundings, and she swears she sees zombies who are talking to her and communicating with her directly, she can't even begin to figure out how to describe it without sounding like a conspiracy theorist. The squirrels didn't have any advice on that either.

Thinking about all of that gave Beth a headache. She decided not to think about it anymore. In the meantime, Beth was being inundated by a treasure trove of sea glass. She found it on walks, in her driveway, piling up in her living room, and in piles outside the sunroom. Her new theory was that the squirrels were gathering it like they would acorns, and she loved it, so she kept filling her jar. It was strange, however. The more she fidgeted with the sea glass, the more her fingers tingled. And she was getting more and more tired. So, she spent even more time sitting on the couch, watching TV, and fidgeting with the sea glass. After Beth spent a few hours of watching TV and listening to the conspiracy theorist stories, the stories started to make more and more sense, and it frightened her. Maybe they weren't conspiracies. Maybe it was the truth. Strange things definitely were happening.

Beth had started wondering if there was a poltergeist in her house, or at least, a mischievous elf who kept moving things. There was nothing major wrong, but a series of annoyances made her wonder. For example, she would put a placemat on the dining room table, lay out the napkin and silverware, and put her beverage glass down on the placemat. Everything would be fine until she returned to the dining room table with her dinner plate of food. She'd sit down, take a sip of her drink, go to put it back down on the placemat, and it was as if the placemat had moved. Inevitably, at least two or three times per meal, her glass would fall off the edge of the placemat. She swore she was doing everything exactly the same way and came to the conclusion that someone or something was moving the placemat while she was sitting there. She couldn't manage to find the edge.

In the meantime, however, she met more people as she walked. All of them were friendly enough, certainly not effusive, but not standoffish. They all were tall and thin with entirely nondescript faces, hair, build, clothing, etc. They were the type of people you'd never be able to identify in a lineup because they looked like generic humans. They had a gray pallor to their skin and their hair was mousey. It wasn't too short. It wasn't too long. They seem to be average. Beth couldn't differentiate among them. That was strange for her, because she used to pride herself on being able to recognize faces and names quite easily.

In the meantime, the world was obsessed with video calls. There were office meetings, webinars, virtual conferences, social gatherings, telemedicine, and many other things that used to be held in person that were now done through the computer. Teenage boys had no problem with this. They were used to being stuck on their computers all day playing games. But the rest of the world felt isolated socially.

Because of these video calls, a strange etiquette emerged. Afraid of being caught undressed, in bed, etc., people put avatars on their screens instead of live video. When live video was important, people dressed from the waist up while remaining in their pajama bottoms or wearing no pants whatsoever. There were many embarrassing examples of people forgetting the video camera was on and they had no pants on as they got up to refill their coffee during a video call. Most video calls had similar dialogue: "Hello, hello, can you hear me?" "We can see you, but we are not hearing anything. You're on mute. Click the picture of the microphone with the red line through it. Take yourself off mute," "Please put yourself on mute. We can hear you crunching potato chips on the call and it's disturbing everyone," "We can hear you, but we can't see you. It looks like you dialed in on your phone. You need to click the video link on the email I sent you so we can see you," and those conversations were for the lucky ones. Other people had to call participants on their landlines to tell them how to get onto the video calls. The zombies, in particular, were completely amused by the lack of technological skill of most humans. Their invasion clearly wasn't going to pose much of a challenge. If humanity couldn't figure out how to do a video call, it certainly couldn't figure out how to undo alien disruptive technology.

Beth and her friends attended virtual happy hours, virtual cooking classes, and virtual book clubs. Beth was puzzled by the concept. Why did she need to have a video screen in her kitchen while she was cooking dinner? Why did she need to cook the meal, the identical meal, that her friends were cooking in their houses — following the same recipe? She was alone in her own house. Couldn't she eat whatever she wanted? She was even more puzzled by the virtual happy hours. Was she supposed to sit by herself and drink alone because someone was on a video call at the same time? Why would she do that? She never understood book clubs to begin with, so a virtual book club was something that stressed her out completely. She loved to read. She loved to think about what she had read. She had no interest in slowing down her reading speed to read slowly enough so the other members of the book club could catch up with her. She found it frustrating because she could go through two or three books in the same time as it took the other members of the book club to read one book. By the time they got around to discussing the first book, she was already done with the third book and couldn't remember anything about the first book. So, it seemed entirely normal to her to not pay attention on these social video calls. She was bored with the fake social interaction. She had plenty of other things to do to keep her busy. Her friends thought otherwise and gave her a hard time. They said she was not paying attention and zoning out. That aggravated her.

On the other hand, it made her happy that she and Jim primarily messaged each other and hadn't yet had a video or telephone/voice interaction. She wouldn't want him to think she wasn't paying attention. In her mind, there wasn't any point in trying to focus on a computer screen, any more than there was a purpose in trying to focus on a TV screen. She'd never been good at that. However, she didn't recognize that she was getting worse at paying attention to and remaining focused on anything.

If anyone had asked her, Beth would've told them how highly organized she was, how focused she was, and she would have put a positive spin on her newly enhanced OCD. She would spend hours upon hours rearranging her stockpiles, her dresser drawers, and her closet. She even spent a full day sorting her sock drawer. Then she became obsessed with the plastic containers in her kitchen. She never seemed to be able to find the matching lid when she put food into the container. Had she been thinking about it or paying attention, she would have matched the lid and the container before she put the food in the container. But, this thought completely evaded her. So, instead, she took every container in the kitchen, and matched the lid. She was mildly surprised at how many lids did not match. At one point, when she moved into the house, she treated herself to a new box of plastic containers with interlocking lids. She has lost many of those lids and had lidless containers. Unwilling to throw out any of the mismatched containers or extra lids, she made a box of misfit containers and put it in the garage. Then she methodically disassembled all of the matching containers and lids, put the lids in one box in her kitchen, and put the lidless containers in another box in the kitchen. This was clearly a poor plan which drove Beth crazy. The next day, she re-sorted the sock drawer and re-matched the containers. At least this time the containers and lids were in the same room.

The sock drawer was never going to be okay, however. Everyone knows that the washing machine and dryer eat socks. It's one of the mysteries of life. No one knows the answer to how one can put two socks into the washing machine and dryer and one comes out. Beth has developed quite an impressive pile of mismatched socks which she has placed on top of her nightstand. Almost daily, she unmatches the socks in the sock drawer and tries to match them with the unmatched socks on the nightstand. She's never successful.

On the other hand, her sea glass collection is progressing extremely well, in her opinion. She is quite successful at finding sea glass in odd locations. She is careful to keep the glass clean and will wash each piece with soap and water at least a few times a week. Her process is quite thorough. She takes all of the sea glass out of the jar, puts it in a colander in the sink, adds soap and water, hand washes each piece, rinses them thoroughly, and then pours the contents of the colander out onto the drying mat on the counter. Then, she takes a soft cloth and hand dries and polishes each piece before putting it back into the jar. It soothes her to do this, even though it makes her tingly, dizzy, and feel off balance. She inevitably stumbles as she brings the jar back and forth to the kitchen and recently, she's come close to dropping the jar a few times. It's easy to blame her clumsiness on not paying attention or on her hands still being soapy and wet. It's the same excuse she uses when she can't open a jar or a container.

6

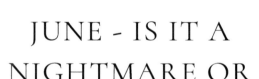

JUNE - IS IT A NIGHTMARE OR REALITY?

Beth continued to find and collect sea glass until her jar was overflowing. She had progressed to a sea glass lamp. Her collection of those beautiful discs still was growing. She was hoping she'd be able to have a pair of matching lamps. It looked like she was well on her way. Watching the sea glass catch the light, both sunlight and from the lamp, made Beth smile. If only she had recognized the danger to her sanity the sea glass posed. The tingling in her arm and leg and the dizziness/headaches were almost constant. Most concerning, however, was her declining ability to recognize the difference between reality and fantasy. Was she awake? Was she dreaming? Was she hallucinating? Was it real?

The road warrior was back. Beth was a scheduled speaker for a 10,000-person conference. She had emailed a copy of her speech to the conference organizer who uploaded the PowerPoint presentation into the conference's computer system. There was a technical team to ensure the presentation would be ready when it was Beth's time to speak. All she had to do was show up and give a presentation she'd done hundreds of times. Because she had both run conferences and been a keynote speaker at meetings where the technology completely failed, she always carried a thumb drive with a copy of her PowerPoint and had a printed hard copy. That way, she could give the speech even if all the technology failed. She'd done it before.

This time, she was walking through the hotel with a stack of papers, some were in folders, some were loose, the pile was awkward, and she was having difficulty balancing the paperwork with her pocketbook and the bag of goodies the conference handed to every meeting attendee. To top it off, she was lost. It was a hotel she'd been in many times, but she couldn't find the meeting rooms. She kept wandering up and down the corridors of the sleeping room areas, ended up at the pool, found the restaurant, but couldn't find the meeting rooms. Even more bizarre there were no elevators and no stairs. Instead, there was a maze of ramps connecting multiple floors and multiple buildings.

At one point she left the convention center by following one of the ramps and ended up in an office building next-door. Then, she couldn't get out of the office building back to the convention center/hotel. She was walking faster and faster up and down these ramps through a maze all while juggling her pile of papers and the two bags. She dropped the papers on the floor and as she bent over to pick them up, the contents of her pocketbook dropped on the floor as well. Time was ticking. Time was moving quickly. Time was moving exponentially faster and faster as she tried to pick her items off the floor. They kept rolling away down the ramp. The papers started flying off the floor and swirling around her like a tornado. The corridor and ramp she was in expanded to be a huge room looking like an old high school gymnasium. Laughing people were pointing at her. She knew she was going to be late for her presentation; everyone was relying on her, and here she was totally lost trying to pick up papers and pens, lipstick, her reading glasses, and all the tchotchkes handed out from the meeting. The tumult went on and on and on.

To make it worse, she desperately had to use the bathroom. She knew she was not going to make it through an hour presentation if she didn't use the bathroom before she went on stage. She finally gathered up most of her belongings, shoved them into the meeting bag, and desperately searched for a bathroom on the way to the meeting room. The first bathroom she went in had no toilets. Every one of the stalls had an out-of-order sign on it. The second bathroom had toilets but no doors on the stalls and the room was full of people, so she wasn't comfortable using those. The third bathroom she found was filthy and she wasn't comfortable using it. It was full of trash, moldy showers, and she didn't even want to know what was on the floor. She still was following all those ramps, faster and faster and more desperately than ever, trying to find the meeting room. She was dizzy, her muscles felt weak, and she bumped into the wall a few times trying to find the bathroom. She never found the bathroom, but she did find a cafeteria that looked generically like any college cafeteria on the planet. She grabbed something to eat, sat down, and realized she was home in her own dining room and the pesky poltergeist hadn't let up for a second. While his favorite thing to do was to move the placemat so her glass fell off of it every night, now he started moving things in the kitchen, and the bathroom, and pretty much every other countertop. Beth would reach for something she saw clearly in front of her and miss it by a couple of inches. Clearly the poltergeist was moving things again.

That night, Beth went to sleep with poltergeists on her mind. A few minutes after dozing off, she realized she had forgotten to message Jim, and she hadn't checked to see if he had messaged her. She got out of bed, turned on the lights, and checked her messages. She had missed more than a dozen from him. As usual, he told her she was beautiful, she was the woman of his dreams, he loved her, and he couldn't wait to see her but he was stuck at work overseas. Sitting in her sunroom and looking out at the stars, it gave her some comfort that they were sleeping beneath the same sky. She liked knowing he could see the same stars she could.

Beth needed the comfort. She was beginning to think something was very wrong. It was as if her brain was testing her mettle. It was challenging her to the point that she was beginning to doubt her sanity.

Often, she was overcome by The Fear. The naked, wild, uncontrolled fear became a being unto itself. Beth would sit bolt upright and scream. She never was sure what had awoken her. "One minute, I'm safe and warm inside my cocoon," she thought. "It's safe, warm, and shimmery silver. And then, it's not." Beth realized she hadn't felt completely safe in a long time. That cocoon made her feel safe, even if for a short time.

Yet, she would wake up screaming. As she tried to make sense of her dream/nightmare, she would remember part of it. She had been safe and warm in her cocoon, then the next thing she knew, the cocoon was being torn open, and her nightmares came alive.

"Run!" her mind screamed. "You can outrun this giant bear that's tearing at you," it urged. "Shit. No, I can't. I'm caught in the cocoon," Beth thought. "It's ripping my cocoon and grabbing for me. What are you supposed to do around bears? Yell? Make myself bigger? Hit it? I can't remember," Beth panicked.

By now, Beth was in a frenzy. "Yell. That's it. I'm going to scream until it goes away. "She let out the most bloodcurdling scream ever. The bear doesn't back down. It's torn Beth's cocoon so her arms and head are exposed, but her legs are caught. The cocoon is trapping her, and the bear is still pulling at her. "Wow. That's strange," Beth thought. "The bear is wearing a pink shirt and pink pants and has purple hands. It's still grabbing at me. I'm terrified!"

Oh no. I think I've wet myself. The bear has literally scared the piss right out of me. Why won't it back down? It's still grabbing at me and tearing the cocoon." Beth couldn't tell if this was a nightmare or real. But the pee running down her leg definitely was real, and she knew it.

"Hitting. That's it. I need to hit that bear until it stops grabbing at me. I gather all my strength and smash that bear right in the chest. Oops. No, I didn't. It jumped away. It doesn't stop. It keeps on tearing at my cocoon. Hey, it freed my feet. Now, I can run!" Beth's thoughts came at alarming speed and were jumbled, but she had no choice but to react and listen to the thoughts in her head.

With superhuman strength, Beth shoved that bear away and knocked it to the ground. It seems stunned as it lies there on the ground, but Beth didn't have time to ponder. She knew she had to get out of there. Beth raced through an opening that had appeared in the wall. It leads directly to... a maze?! "There's a bear behind me, and a maze in front of me?" Beth was incredulous. "With all the wild adventures in my life, and I've been around a long time, I can't say I remember a situation like this," Beth thought to herself. Beth glanced behind her at the destruction of her cocoon and the pink-clothed bear slowly rising off the floor. Clearly, she had knocked the wind out of it. "Can't say I'm sorry — clearly it deserved to be punished for destroying my cocoon and attacking me!" Beth looked for another way out.

Beth found the front door, and she ran. She ran faster than she's ever run. She didn't know where she was running, but she knew she needed to run. She was so engrossed in her own thoughts that she didn't realize she had been running in circles around her house, and she didn't notice the silver RV hovering on the street behind her. She noticed her view of the stars was suddenly obscured by fog, and she was surprised at the sudden cold breeze coming through the closed sliding glass doors in her sunroom. She didn't know how she got back into her sunroom. She also didn't understand why she was freezing cold. It was June, after all, and usually it was hot in D.C.

The next thing Beth knew, her sliding glass door opened, and one of her neighbors was standing there. For the life of her, she couldn't tell exactly which neighbor it was. He seemed like a nameless, faceless person with no real identifying facial characteristics. He had mousy brown hair, was tall, thin, and she had a vague recollection of seeing him before but had no idea who he was. She looked at his face and couldn't see anything. There was no recognition. Clearly, he was dressed better for the weather than she was. He was wearing a bulky blue sweater, and it made sense since he was standing in the cold fog. Beth was wearing her usual summer sleepwear... A Red Sox T-shirt and underpants. Fortunately, the shirt was big enough and long enough to cover anything she would have been embarrassed to have her neighbor see. Her neighbor reached out his hand for her, and for some reason she still doesn't understand, she took it. His hand was cold and clammy. Yet, for some reason, she felt safe.

"It's a beautiful night," he said. "I thought you'd like to take a ride with me. I saw your light was on, so I figured you were still up." Beth didn't know what to say, so she didn't say anything. Instead, she followed him out of the sunroom across her backyard and into the RV. Inside, the RV was incredibly high-tech. It was nothing like the old-fashioned RVs which were decorated in linoleum and Formica. This was glistening with shiny, sleek surfaces, ergonomically comfortable-looking furniture, and was well-stocked with Diet Coke® and pretzels. Beth immediately felt at home. It bothered her that she couldn't remember exactly which neighbor this was, but still she felt safe. As they drove down the street, she was impressed by the smoothness of the ride. Her neighbor managed to miss the big dip in the road that everyone else hit. He went over it smoothly. Every time Beth went over the dip in the road, she was worried she was going to lose an axle or tire on her car.

"Make yourself comfortable," her neighbor said. "Let's go on a road trip."

By this point, Beth had lost track of time but realized she had gotten into a strange neighbor's RV and didn't have any pants on. She also didn't have any shoes on. She was in a T-shirt, underpants, and nonskid socks. She didn't have her phone with her, she didn't have her wallet with her, she hadn't locked up her house; in fact, the back slider to the sunroom was wide open. So she said, "Thanks, but can we please go back to my house? I'd like to change my clothes and grab my pocketbook."

The neighbor replied, "Why don't you check the closet in the bedroom at the back of the RV? Maybe there are some clothes there you'd enjoy. I always keep the closet well-stocked because I never know what the weather's going to be like around here. And," he continued, "don't worry about needing your wallet or anything like that, this adventure is my treat!"

Rising from her seat, being careful to make sure her T-shirt covered the fact that she was not wearing any pants, Beth made her way to the back of the RV into the closet. While her neighbor had said he had plenty of clothes, she was impressed at the selection. She found a pair of navy stretch pants in the perfect size and was pleased to see they matched her T-shirt. Exploring further, she found a Red Sox sweatshirt that also matched her T-shirt, so she put that on over her T-shirt. She had just realized she wasn't wearing a bra, and she was immediately self-conscious. Just as she wished she had been wearing a bra when she left her house, she noticed a bureau.

She'd already lucked out finding pants and a sweatshirt that were her style, color, and size, she mused, so why not see if there was a bra in the drawer? There were a few brand-new ones with the tags still on them, and all of them were the style, size, and color she favored. Next to the bras was a pack of her favorite socks she always wore under her sneakers when she went for a walk. She hurriedly got dressed. She was mildly surprised when she looked at the floor at the foot of the bed where she was sitting to get dressed and found a brand-new pair of her favorite sneakers. They, too, still had the tags on them. She should have been surprised at the attention to detail for what she thought was an impromptu ride, but for some reason, it felt entirely normal to her.

Fully dressed, and completely comfortable, Beth moved into the passenger seat at the front of the RV. Her neighbor was in the driver's seat as she had left him. He looked her up and down and nodded his head in satisfaction. She buckled her seatbelt, thanked him for being so generous, and then asked him where they were headed. He said nothing and pointed to the ground. Beth noticed the RV was gently rising above the street getting higher and higher above the treetops until they were hovering at about the same height as a helicopter would. The difference was she was sitting in an RV and the movement was more gliding and gentler than the choppiness of a helicopter. She was flying. Like the wish everyone in D.C. has: to rise above the traffic and fly to wherever you needed to be. That wish was Beth's reality.

Gliding over the highways on a peaceful calm night, Beth noticed fog all around her that would clear away as she flew through it. Her view was entirely unobstructed, and it was gorgeous. She'd always loved visiting the monuments in downtown D.C. at night, and tonight was no exception. She and her neighbor glided over the White House, around the top of the Washington Monument and the Lincoln Memorial, and then flew back over the Martin Luther King Memorial and the Jefferson Memorial before heading to Capitol Hill. The monuments at night are gorgeous. The lighting is beautiful; there's a stillness to the city, and a sense of peace. Briefly, Beth wondered why there were no fighter jets coming after her because clearly she was flying in restricted airspace. But she allowed herself to suspend her disbelief and enjoy the ride. In the blink of an eye, she saw the Statue of Liberty and then the lights of Manhattan.

Then she saw the ocean. They flew over great expanses of the ocean, and Beth was mesmerized by the details of the waves and the boats below even though there was fog all around the RV. Again, it was as if the RV could cut through the fog so she could see everything below her clearly. As she was pondering this, she realized she was flying over the Kremlin. She had always wanted to go to Eastern Europe; she stared out the window like an eager tourist. The RV flew closer to the ground, and she could see the statue of Lenin. Not far away, she saw a soaring half-arch. She'd never seen that. Her companion turned to her and said it was the monument to the "conquerors of space." Then they circled Red Square. She had expected to see the stereotypically Russian historical buildings, but she was completely surprised by a tall, gleaming, metallic building that looked roughly like the double helix of DNA. It was fascinating seeing the juxtaposition of old and new Moscow. As soon as they were there, they were gone.

Beth looked down again, and they were in London. There was Big Ben. There was the London Bridge. The next thing Beth knew, she was flying over the pyramids of Egypt. She'd always wanted to go see the pyramids, so she was particularly thrilled. Recognizing the ridiculousness of her next thought, Beth wished she had had her cell phone so she could take pictures of everything she was seeing to post them on social media. But without her phone, she was instead forced to live in the moment and enjoy what she was seeing without worrying about posting it.

In the blink of an eye, they flew past Jerusalem and the Wailing Wall. Literally seconds later, they were at the Sydney Opera House. As soon as she saw the Golden Gate Bridge in San Francisco, she knew she was almost home. Normally, it was a six-hour flight on an airplane, but clearly this RV had some good speed on it.

Beth was amazed when the RV made a U-turn around Mount Rushmore, flew back to the desert, and landed in front of a dilapidated diner with plastic alien sculptures outside of it. She nearly dissolved in a fit of giggles. After seeing the magnificence of things around her earlier that evening, it was a letdown to land in front of plastic, cartoonlike aliens. Her neighbor turned to her and said, "I've always wanted to stop here. Let's get something to eat. My treat." He claimed to have seen this particular diner on TV and was intrigued. Hence, this particular stop on the round-the-world road trip.

Beth was amused when they walked from the RV which her neighbor had parked in the parking lot next to all the "regular" cars and RVs as if they had driven there from down the street. Then, a strange object caught her eye. It was a payphone. She hadn't seen one of those in twenty years. She had to see if it worked. Much to her surprise, when she lifted the receiver, it had a dial tone. She searched for the coin slot and then realized she didn't have any. It was okay, though. The change slot had been covered up with duct tape. She had a dial tone, so she thought she would try to make a phone call. As her fingers hovered over the buttons, she froze. She realized she didn't know anyone's phone number. She would tell her phone to call someone, and as long as they were in her contact list, the phone dialed it. She hadn't remembered anyone's phone number in decades. She vaguely remembered that sometimes one would have to dial a one before the number for long distance, and when she was a child, there weren't any area codes. She had a flashback to childhood. In those days, the phone company used to be able to tell you the time and weather if you dialed WE6-1234. How she remembered that she'll never know.

Of course, that's been happening more and more to her lately. She could remember her university ID number, the combination to her high school gym locker, but was completely unable to recall the password to her computer. Sighing to herself about how she's clearly gotten older than she wishes to admit, she decides to dial WE6-1234. She smiled to herself as she started to dial. First of all, when the phone system started using area codes, they changed the WE6 to 936. She had forgotten that. Fortunately, she remembered that as her finger was hovering over the pushbuttons, because the phone was so old the keys were faded. She could, however, remember the positions of where the keys should be on the phone, so she punched away. And nothing happened. She tried again and again. It never dawned on her that the problem wasn't necessarily with the phone, but there probably was never a need to dial for time and temperature anymore, and the number she was trying to reach didn't work. She was incredibly frustrated she couldn't make the phone work, and she should have realized she knew her own phone number and could have left a message. But she didn't. Sensing her frustration, her neighbor tapped her on her shoulder and motioned toward the restaurant.

They went inside. It was a stereotypical greasy spoon with all-day breakfast, hamburgers, fried everything, and homemade desserts. Looking at the menu, Beth thought the theme of the restaurant should have been "heart attack on a plate." She loves patty melts, grilled cheese and bacon or tomato sandwiches, and things like that. However, she could not justify a triple-decker patty melt wrapped in bacon and deep fried. She was mesmerized by all of the ways bacon could be incorporated into a menu. While Beth normally didn't eat pork, for some reason, the occasional piece of crispy bacon was okay, although she preferred turkey bacon. She knew better than to ask for turkey bacon in a place like this. She also had a deep-seated hatred of all things mayonnaise. She knew trying to special order something without mayonnaise was not going to be effective here. At least that narrowed down some of her choices.

Much to her horror, however, the waitress handed her a chicken sandwich with mayonnaise and bacon. Beth has a deep aversion to chicken, and as mentioned earlier, she hates mayonnaise. The waitress winked at her and said, "Just kidding. May I suggest the grilled cheese sandwich with tomato and bacon… It's excellent!" Beth breathed a sigh of relief, happy with that suggestion, and asked for a side of homemade potato chips and a large Diet Coke®. Her neighbor stared at the menu like he had never eaten before. He ordered the full lumberjack breakfast with bacon, ham, sausage, home fried potatoes, eggs over easy, and a side of pancakes. Then, he spied another waitress carrying a Belgian waffle piled high with ice cream, whipped cream, hot fudge, and strawberries. He asked for that, too. The portions at this restaurant were huge. Each plate was the size of a steering wheel of a car and heaped with food. He must have consumed a pound of bacon, a pound of potatoes, half a dozen eggs, and everything else that he ordered — and doused it all in a whole bottle of syrup. He washed it down with an entire pot of coffee. While Beth had taken the world tour by a flying RV in stride, watching her thin neighbor eat all of that food threw her for a loop. "Life is totally unfair," she thought. "He at least could gain weight eating like that… If there were any justice in the world, he would weigh a thousand pounds." But he didn't.

As they walked back to the RV after their gorge-fest with her neighbor carrying a huge bag of alien-themed tchotchkes from the gift shop, her neighbor asked if she could spare a few more minutes so he could show her two more things before they returned home. Wired from the Diet Coke® and too many free refills, she was thrilled to say yes. Once she was safely buckled back into her seat in the RV, her neighbor slowly drove down the road in front of the diner. Surprisingly, Beth felt every bump and dip on the road. It appeared they no longer were hovering but were driving. Then she saw signs reading "Area 51" and "Extraterrestrial Highway" with arrows pointing in the direction they were headed. They reached a menacing-looking fence topped with barbed wire, and clearly electrified. "Federal Property. Do Not Enter" signs were posted all over the fence. Her neighbor reached over and pushed a button on the dashboard of the RV. And then, he drove straight ahead as the fence dissolved around them. Once inside the compound, he told Beth to sit tight for a minute as he went outside the RV. She heard the RV hum and vibrate. She looked outside her window and saw the base of the RV surrounded by fog. She had this odd sense that her neighbor was refueling the RV, and the fog was an integral part. Part of what, she didn't know.

Her neighbor had clearly finished whatever he had set out to do. He got back into his seat, buckled up, and the RV lifted straight up in the air and started flying. He acted quite amused and immensely proud of himself. Then, unable to contain himself, he burst out laughing. He looked at Beth, and once he stopped his hysterical laughter, he apologized for not being able to share the joke. Matter-of-factly, he said she wouldn't understand. She accepted that. By now, she was much more interested in where the RV was going. This time, it wasn't flying over land or oceans, it was going straight up toward the stars. They reached the international space station. As they circled the space station, her neighbor waved at the astronauts, and flashed them a handwritten sign that said, "Hi!" And then the RV headed back to Earth.

Minutes later, Beth was home and back in her own bed. She was so tired she fell asleep in her new sweatshirt and sweatpants. At least she took off her shoes.

Beth slept so soundly, even with the TV on, that she missed the news reports about hordes of people suddenly getting well and recovering from having been zombies in Washington, D.C., New York, Moscow, London, Sydney, and San Francisco. All of them had some pneumonia, apparently the first sign of becoming a zombie, yet they all were suddenly and miraculously cured.

7

JULY - THE MOUSE ARRIVES

The next month started innocently enough. A few months ago, Beth had found a dog cookie in the middle of her floor outside her closet in her bedroom. It was strange because while she always had treats for dogs in the kitchen cabinet, she herself did not own a dog. None of the dogs she knew would ever take a cookie and leave it somewhere else in the house. They all would eat it as quickly as they could grab it while standing in the kitchen. Furthermore, she couldn't figure out how a cookie could get out of the cabinet by itself. She was puzzled.

She didn't think any more about it until today. She was sitting in the dining room when, out of the corner of her eye she swore she saw a little creature run out from behind the refrigerator, skirt the edge of the kitchen cabinet, and disappear. She wasn't sure she had seen anything, so she blinked her eyes a few times and went back to sorting her mail. After thinking about it, she decided finding the cookie in the middle of the floor and seeing the little creature might be related. Maybe she had a mouse in the house. She was more curious than alarmed since she hadn't seen the mouse completely yet. That changed later that night. She was in the bathroom, sitting on the toilet to be exact, when she started coughing uncontrollably. In between coughs, she leaned over to get toilet paper to blow her nose and saw a mouse sitting on the bathmat on its hind legs with its front paws in a praying motion, looking right at her. The mouse was more curious than afraid, and she had the feeling the mouse was checking to make sure she was okay. It had appeared out of nowhere. As quickly as it appeared, it disappeared. One of her favorite books as a child had featured a mouse adopted by a family. The mouse sitting on her bathmat made her smile and think of that book. Still with a smile on her face, she finished up in the bathroom and went to bed.

A few nights later, she was lying in her bed watching TV when she saw a mouse calmly walk into her bedroom. It was not scurrying, it was not afraid; it strolled in as if it belonged there. It stopped and looked at her, and she swore it gave her a wave. Then it walked under the dresser and she didn't see it again. This became a nightly ritual. The mouse would come in, wave goodnight, and go to sleep under her bureau. Every night she said goodnight to the mouse. Every morning, the mouse would come out from under the bureau, wave goodbye, and head out to do whatever it is mice do during the day.

Beth was confused because she thought mice were nocturnal animals, and this one slept at night in her bedroom and left to go to work during the day. As time went on, the mouse stopped longer and longer before he went under the bureau to go to sleep. She talked to him, and he didn't run away. In fact, he would sit patiently looking at her as if waiting for her to speak. She found herself looking forward to their conversations. He was a good listener even if he was not particularly talkative. Over time, however, the mouse started to speak to her. Surprisingly, he was a good conversationalist. He was kind, funny, and explained that the world was getting strange outside, and he would appreciate it if she would allow him to rent the space under the bureau. Since he was kind, and Beth welcomed the company, she told him he didn't need to pay rent but he was more than welcome to stay there. Their evening conversations became a ritual. It was one of her favorite parts of the night. Talking to the mouse calmed her restlessness.

Rearranging her bureau drawers also calmed her restlessness. She wanted to make sure she didn't disturb the mouse that lived underneath, so she moved on to rearranging her closets. It became a nightly ritual that lasted for hours. Talking to the mouse while she rearranged closets calmed her down, usually.

One night, however, Beth was particularly restless. She often was restless, and in more poetic moments, she would refer to this restlessness as wanderlust. That was one of the reasons she was so excited to take that world tour with her neighbor in the middle of the night. Tonight would have been a good night to repeat that experience. But she couldn't remember which of her neighbors had taken her on that tour. All she knew was it was one of her thin, nondescript neighbors with mousy brown hair who favored navy blue sweaters. That wasn't a lot to go on. Sighing to herself, she tried to settle down on the big, hot pink, throne-like chair in her sunroom and stare out the window.

Later that night, she felt as though she were floating. When she looked down, she still was sitting in the big pink chair, but she wasn't in her sunroom anymore. Her pink chair was in the back seat of an old-fashioned fighter jet. There was a pilot in the front, and she was in her chair in the backseat directly behind him. She felt out of control because she couldn't see past the pilot to see what was in front of her. It was frightening. Not knowing where they were going, how to get there, or if they would hit anything in front of them, Beth got more agitated. She felt totally out of control, and hated it. In the back of her mind, she was grateful she had her pocketbook strapped across her chest, because at least she knew she'd have her telephone with her.

She was totally disoriented about place and time, and found that incredibly disconcerting, because in the back of her mind she knew she had a presentation coming up. She always would email the presentation to herself so it was on her phone, and put that in her wallet, and carry a paper copy with her, just in case she lost something. Today, sitting in the back of that fighter jet, feeling helpless and scared, she had something else to worry about. She realized that all along, her pattern of backup upon backup to not lose a presentation had one fatal flaw. If anybody stole her pocketbook, they'd likely have both her phone and the thumb drive. This was what she obsessed about. And then, the airplane landed safely on the sidewalk in front of a large, beautiful hotel. There were books stacked in the window of the hotel lobby facing the street. And, in the same window, there was a sign with Beth's face on it. She realized the hotel was promoting her book signing. Those were her books. She looked more closely at the pocketbook strapped across her chest and realized it wasn't her pocketbook after all. It was a makeup case. There was nothing in it except eyeshadow, lipstick, and mascara. She was without her phone, without her thumb drive, without a speech, and without the copy of her book she had highlighted and marked with sticky notes.

Then, she looked down at her clothes and realized she was wearing the same sweatpants and Red Sox sweatshirt she had been wearing on her previous tour in the RV. This was no way to present herself at a book signing. Looking up at the hotel, she realized she was at the Plaza Hotel in New York City. It is a high-end hotel in a high-end city. She guessed she was probably the only person in the entire area who was wearing sweats. And she most certainly, given the rivalry between the Boston Red Sox and New York Yankees, was the only person wearing a Red Sox sweatshirt. Now was a good time to panic.

Unsure of what to do next, Beth allowed the doorman to assist her out of the airplane. Looking back at her big pink chair that should be in the sunroom in her house, she saw a bookbag lying across the seat. It had a replica of her book cover on it. It gave her a glimmer of hope that she might have packed her phone, the thumb drive, or her marked-up copy of her book. The doorman reached back into the plane and handed her the bookbag. No one seemed to be surprised that an airplane had landed on the sidewalk in front of a fancy hotel in the middle of Manhattan. Holding her head high, grasping her bookbag, Beth followed the doorman into the hotel. The hotel manager greeted them and said, "We've been expecting you. Your suite is right this way." He brought Beth to a magnificent suite. And there, much to Beth's delight, were two rolling racks of clothes. "Your publicist sent the clothes over, and your stylist is on her way," said the hotel manager. "In the meantime, the spa downstairs is ready to do your hair and makeup." And there, on the desk, was a copy of Beth's book, a paper copy of her speech, and the thumb drive.

Beth was so relieved her team had taken care of everything that she didn't notice that as the airplane took off from the sidewalk, a mist followed behind it. Nor did she notice it made sure to circle the entire city before it headed back to Washington.

That night, giddy from an incredibly successful book signing, Beth couldn't sleep. Settling in among the fluffy pillows in an oversized bed in her beautiful suite in a luxury hotel in Manhattan, Beth tossed and turned and fidgeted. Turning on the TV, she was flabbergasted by what she saw. No matter what channel, the only thing available was the news. The newscasters were of all shapes and sizes, all ethnicities, and clearly reporting from all over the world. In voices and tones that barely concealed their panic, they talked about the need for worldwide testing. Beth wasn't sure why they were talking about testing and for what? Reading? Writing? STEM? STEAM? Beth started obsessing over the words "stem" versus "steam." She couldn't remember what was politically correct anymore. Beth hoped the reporters were talking about testing people to ensure they weren't morons and could think for themselves. That hope was short-lived, however. It seemed as though the testing was related to this strange mist descending over major cities throughout the world or testing for zombies who were causing the citizens there to act like idiots. There were photos and videos of strangely groomed and oddly dressed people cramming into rooms and dancing, and yelling, and singing, packed in so tightly there was barely an inch between people. And the reporters started screaming into the cameras, "Stay at home! Stay at home! For G-d's sake, stay at home!" And no one listened.

From their outpost on Mars, the aliens sat in their RVs, looked down at Earth, and laughed. They couldn't believe the humans would panic about toilet paper, bottled water, Jell-O®, Chinese food, and cookies, but that they didn't recognize the real danger was the zombies and that the fog would save them. The aliens had been hoping for a good thriller show, and instead they felt they were handed a Laurel and Hardy routine. So they upped their game. This show needed a good plot twist. The aliens wondered if they should let humanity suffer at the hands of the zombies, if they should tell the humans that they, the aliens, had the antidote for the zombie apocalypse, or watch the show play out. They decided humanity would provide its own plot twist. For the time being, they did nothing. It irked them, though, that the perceptions of aliens were so negative and most of humanity assumed the aliens were trying to destroy Earth, when in this particular case, they were trying to save the humans from themselves and the zombies. The aliens needed a better PR agency.

The zombies were experts at social media. They planted stories that appealed to human greed and selfishness. There were hundreds of social media posts about how "your" individual rights were being taken away. Every time a scientist spoke up about zombies threatening humanity, zombies would post more "news" stories about how the scientists were spreading "fake news." And many humans believed the zombies. The zombies and the aliens were curious to see how far humans would follow absurdity. Their last real attempt had been in 1939 with a radio program based on H. G. Wells and *The War of the Worlds*. The ensuing panic was quite amusing for the aliens and the zombies. At that time, the world only had the radio to rely on, not the instant video and social media distribution it did in 2020. One of the most disappointing features for the aliens was the total lack of panic when they released the fog in major cities throughout the world. At least back then, the radio story of the Martians releasing poison gas in New York caused some panic. The modern-day response was ho-hum, to say the least.

The continuing unrest promoted through social media provided some entertainment value to the aliens and the zombies, but not enough to keep them completely occupied. They felt the ongoing zombie apocalypse was the equivalent of a human TV show being in reruns. It was interesting, but not worth becoming immersed in. Searching for more excitement, the aliens stopped hanging out at their outpost on

Mars and moved to the greasy diner outside Area 51. The food was better. And, no one batted an eyelash at a room full of nondescript tall thin beings with mousy brown hair and blue sweaters hanging out with zombies. The aliens and the zombies looked more "normal" than some of the humans, at least to some of the human observers, that is. While the zombies were trying to take over humanity, and the aliens were trying to save it, they had formed an alliance solely for entertainment purposes. The humans certainly provided enough entertainment. The aliens and zombies smiled to themselves as they watched the TVs strewn throughout the diner. Every channel featured human unrest. Accusations of government conspiracies, fake news, and general temper tantrum behavior by adults filled the channels. The zombies and the aliens placed bets on the upcoming antics of the humans. It made the game more interesting, after all.

Beth knew none of the background of the zombies versus aliens. All she saw was the behavior of her fellow humans. It stressed her out. There had been so many strange things going on in her life recently she couldn't process one more thing. With that thought, she leaned back against the pillows, closed her eyes, and tried to sleep. She wasn't sure if she had slept or not, because the next thing she realized was she was sitting in her big pink chair in her sunroom and wearing sweats and a Red Sox sweatshirt. The TV was on in her bedroom, and the news reporters were screaming, "Stay-at-home! Stay-at-home!"

She was completely and utterly discombobulated. She would have felt much better texting Jim, or messaging him, but once again, she couldn't find her phone. It must have been the poltergeist. She turned on both of her sea glass lamps and hoped the light would scare off the poltergeist. It didn't. It made her tingly, dizzy, and disoriented. She was too tired to do anything about it, though. Most importantly, however, she still hadn't made the connection.

The mouse was worried. He had never seen her quite this bad. She didn't even bother arranging her closets or talking to him. She mumbled to herself about a poltergeist and thrashed around while dozing on her big pink chair. She never even went to bed.

8

AUGUST - THE POLTERGEIST IS MERCILESS

The poltergeist was getting entirely out of hand. Beth spent more and more of her time trying to find things that weren't where she knew she had put them. At first, she thought the poltergeist moved things, like it moved her placemat on her table. But it seems to have escalated its game. Now it's moving entire objects out of her sight line. For example, she always kept a pair of shoes next to her bed. She's kept shoes next to her bed for decades. It didn't matter which house she was in; she started that habit in her college dorm when the fire alarms used to go off on a regular basis. Having been caught twice with no shoes nearby, she changed her habit and kept a pair of shoes next to her bed. College was a long time ago, so this is a long-time habit. Yet, suddenly, she can never find her shoes. Clearly, the poltergeist has moved them.

Apparently, the poltergeist also is amused by her keys. She has one keychain with her house keys and her car key on it. The keychain is a pink Converse high-top sneaker. It's about 1" x 2" x 3" long. It's not easy to lose it. But the poltergeist moves it on a regular basis. Since she's moved into this house, Beth has kept that keychain on the kitchen counter near where she drops her pocketbook. Yesterday, she found the keys in the refrigerator.

At first, she thought someone was breaking into her house and stealing her "stuff," but she always found it, just in bizarre places. It's clear to her the poltergeist has a sense of humor. It seems to take great pleasure in moving her TV remotes, the remotes that raise and lower her bed, her keys, her sunglasses, and occasionally, her shoes. But most annoying is that it keeps moving her cans of Diet Coke®. She will go to the refrigerator, take out a can of Diet Coke®, open it, and put it down next to her computer, for example. She'll get up from her desk, go to the bathroom, realize she's thirsty, go to the refrigerator, take out a Diet Coke®, and bring it back to put it down next to her computer. She'll vaguely remember having done that earlier in the day, but when she looks, there isn't a Diet Coke® next to the computer. Yet, strangely enough, she may find a mostly full, yet opened, can in the sunroom next to her chair and telephone.

Beth has taken to yelling at the poltergeist when she can't find something. While the poltergeist doesn't answer her, Alexa and Siri do. At least Alexa normally has some semi-helpful advice. Beth alternates between yelling at the poltergeist for moving the stuff and asking Alexa where her stuff is. Recently, however, Beth has become disconcerted by voices talking to each other in her house. Sometimes, these conversations don't even involve her. It seems as though Alexa, Siri, her TV, and her computer are talking to each other behind her back. She has walked into conversations between her iPhone and her iPad where they say to each other, "I don't understand. Can you say that again?" And the other device repeats it. Or, she'll be watching TV, and Alexa will comment on something she heard on TV. It's even stranger when Beth dictates a message to Jim and Siri or Alexa answers back.

Sometimes Beth thinks she's losing her mind. But it's difficult to tell whether the world is going crazy or she is. Maybe it's both.

Regardless of whether Beth is losing her mind, or the world is going crazy, she is completely exhausted. Beth isn't sleeping well at night, is exhausted during the day, and can't concentrate. The other day, she wanted to make eggs and toast for breakfast. She took out the frying pan and put it on the stove. She went to the refrigerator, opened the door, and stared. She completely forgot why she opened the refrigerator. The refrigerator, quite helpfully, started beeping, raising the alarm that she had kept the door open too long. So she shut the door. She turned around and saw the frying pan on the stove. That's right! She remembered she wanted to make scrambled eggs. She opened the refrigerator door, found the eggs, took them out, and put them on the counter next to the stove. The refrigerator beeped at her again since she clearly hadn't shut the door all the way. As she opened the refrigerator door, intending to slam it to make sure it was shut tightly, she realized the milk and butter were still in the refrigerator. She took them out and made sure to tightly shut the refrigerator door this time. She whisked the eggs and milk in a bowl, added butter in a pan, and waited for the butter to melt so she could put the eggs in the pan and scramble them.

After what seemed like an eternity, and the butter still was not melting at all in the pan, Beth got aggravated. She decided to give up on the eggs entirely. Then she hunted for bread to make toast. Gratefully, she spotted it on the counter. She put some slices in the toaster, turned it on, and listened to it click away as it began toasting her bread. That's when she looked back at the stovetop and recognized she hadn't ever turned the stovetop on which is why the pan still was cold and the butter hadn't melted. Feeling stupid and frustrated, she turned on the stovetop, heated up the butter, added the eggs, scrambled them, took the toast out of the toaster, buttered it, and had a great breakfast. Since she had had so much difficulty making breakfast that morning, she was paranoid she had left the stove or the toaster on. She kept checking obsessively.

Of course, the inevitable did happen later that week. She did leave the stovetop on and the eggs and butter caught fire and burned. She's lucky she didn't burn the house down. It scared her so much she stopped cooking. Instead, she chose food that could be eaten cold or heated in the microwave. She knew enough to be afraid. In a strange way, that fear became comforting because she was so afraid of doing something dangerous that she followed the fear and took fewer risks. It comforted her that she might not necessarily do something extremely dangerous like accidentally burn down her house. Other times, she was afraid her fear was making her paranoid. Either way, she was afraid.

"Afraid" was a word she was using more often. "The Fear," which used to come out at night, followed her wherever she went. She couldn't snap herself out of it. She became obsessed with things she was afraid of like snakes, losing things, forgetting things, being lost, people watching her, people recognizing she was an imposter, and fearing they were imposters. The list went on and on. Today, she couldn't shake the feeling that she was late for a college class. There was a final exam, she hadn't ever attended the class, she hadn't studied, and she didn't even know where the class was located. She knew she had to get there. Fortunately, today was one of the days where she could find her shoes. She put them on, opened the door of her house, and left to go to class. Of course, she couldn't find her keys to lock up, so she left the front door unlocked. Since she couldn't find her keys, she couldn't drive anywhere. All she could do was walk to campus. Unfortunately, she couldn't remember where the campus was or how to get there. She kept walking and looking for the campus, looking for her professor, or looking for anything at all familiar. After wandering for what seemed like hours, by some miracle, she ended up back in her neighborhood. She let herself back into her house and collapsed into the big pink chair in her sunroom.

She was glad to be back in familiar surroundings, but terrified she still was late for her class and was going to fail the final exam. The sun was setting, she was comfortable in her chair, yet she was still panicked. She tried to relax to see if she could remember what class she was late for, who the professor was, or any detail. As she tried to relax, the pictures in her mind got more and more terrifying. She had found the professor, but she couldn't quite get to him because his office was full of venomous snakes. The snakes were crawling everywhere. The floor was covered, the chairs were covered, and she could hear them hissing at her. They slithered up her pant legs, and they were mocking her.

She could hear the hissing and understand it as clear as if it were in English. "You're going to fail," they said. "You don't remember how to do calculus," they said. "You can't remember anything, but that doesn't even matter because you didn't know anything to begin with."

Terrified, she ran up and down the hills of her college campus searching for the correct room. She didn't know how she got to the college campus. It was 1500 miles away and a lifetime ago since she had been there. Faster and faster she ran, getting more frightened as time went by. If she didn't pass calculus class, she wasn't going to graduate from college, and if she didn't graduate from college, she was a fraud, and everyone was going to find out she was a fraud, and she couldn't remember anything, and people were going to think she was stupid, and... And The Fear took over. Frenzied, and in a complete panic, she jumped out of her pink chair, ran out the front door of her house, and ran down the street again. Destination unknown, again. She didn't know where she needed to be, but she knew she needed to get there.

She ran until she couldn't run anymore and finally collapsed on a bench. Exhausted, terrified, and completely lost, she burst into tears. It was at that moment her neighbor pulled up in his silver RV, opened the door and said, "Come on in, you're safe." There were other people in the RV, some of them tall, thin, nondescript with mousy brown hair, and others who were more vibrant although a bit dusty. Beth could only think of the phrase "ashes to ashes, dust to dust." She didn't have much experience with zombies, so she didn't recognize them. Her neighbor, still buckled into the driver's seat of the RV, turned to the other people in the RV and said, "She's one of the good ones. There's a reason she's still here, and we need to make sure she's safe." Beth had no idea who was in the RV. She felt safe. She couldn't remember who was driving the RV, but she vaguely remembered seeing him before, and most importantly, he was not the scary professor surrounded by snakes. She settled back in her seat and relaxed.

When the RV pulled into her driveway, Beth was shocked at how beautiful the walkway from her driveway to her front door looked. The whole walkway was covered in glistening worry stones of assorted sizes, sparkling sea glass, and moon stones. They glistened in the moonlight and appeared entirely magical. While they varied in size, they all were smooth, round, and disc-shaped, with a thumbprint on the top. She finally realized why the shape looked familiar. They looked like thumbprint cookies, yet they were made of stone and sea glass. She realized she could not gather all of these up and make even more matching lamps, so she admired their beauty and walked into the house. She had a vague sensation of being off balance both physically and mentally, dragging her right arm and leg, and feeling a tingling throughout her body. She wasn't worried, however, she felt she was getting some power from the stones.

Her pleasure at seeing the beauty of the magical stones as she walked into her house was quite short-lived. She was flabbergasted when she walked into her living room and realized the poltergeist had not only moved her prized possessions, but it had replaced them with fakes. Her crystal vases, for example, were slightly off. They still were on her glass display table, and others still were in her display cabinet, but they didn't seem right. They looked counterfeit. Beth was reminded of the counterfeit pocketbooks one could buy on the streets of New York City; to the casual observer, they looked fine, but to someone who knows, they were clearly fake. This is exactly what happened to Beth's vases. She was horrified. First, she had no idea how someone, even the poltergeist, had managed to switch out her crystal so quickly. Second, she had expensive crystal, and it was rendered valueless. In a panic, she looked for other items of value. She was horrified to find that even items with no monetary value but tons of sentimental value, like her grandmother's menorah, also had been replaced. It was obvious to her that someone had broken into the house, or the poltergeist had replaced the objects himself. She yelled for the mouse to ask him if he had seen anything. He came running to see what was wrong but was puzzled as Beth pointed out the objects she thought were counterfeit.

Beth was hot, she was tired, she was terrified, and she felt violated. Her euphoria at seeing all the beautiful sea glass and moon stones was long gone. She couldn't handle any more. Her brain shut down and she collapsed into bed.

The next morning, Beth woke up and immediately went into her living room to see if anything had changed. The crystal still was counterfeit. Afraid to look, Beth walked over to the shelf containing the items that were most important to her; the objects that had no financial worth but were of extreme sentimental value. She remembered that today, August 31, would have been her grandfather's birthday, were he still alive. She had inherited a silver shoe-shaped pincushion from his mother, her great-grandmother. She couldn't bear to see if anything had happened to it, particularly on his birthday. With trembling hands, she reached out to touch it, and promptly dropped it on the floor. Fortunately, it was relatively indestructible, and it was fine from the fall. As she picked it up from the floor, she heard a voice in her head, clear as if someone were standing next to her, and the voice said, "It's okay. This is real." And she was relieved.

It was strange that hearing her great-grandmother's voice while touching the pincushion should comfort Beth. After all, she was hearing voices from beyond the grave during a zombie apocalypse. On some level, though, she understood why some people weren't afraid of the zombies. In fact, they may have been comforting; loved ones who had passed away who came back to life. Beth gladly took the sense of comfort wherever she could find it.

In moments of clarity over the past eight months, she had been afraid she was losing her mind, and she was terrified. But she had the feeling that at least someone was watching over her. She started to reach out more to people who had passed away. Much to her surprise and joy, she was able to see them, hear them, and talk to them as if they were right in the room with her. To Beth, the timing of all of this made sense. It almost was Rosh Hashanah, and of course her relatives and friends who had passed away were watching over her. She wasn't surprised when they all joined her in her car as she went to the Dunkin' Donuts drive-through to get some iced coffee.

9

SEPTEMBER - ROSH HASHANAH, THE START OF A NEW YEAR

August ended and with September came a new beginning. *Rosh Hashanah, the Jewish New Year was in September this year. Since the Jewish holidays follow the Jewish calendar, it does not always fall in the same month on the Western calendar. But, this year the holiday was in September. Rosh Hashanah* commemorates the creation of the world. Rosh Hashanah is the beginning of the Days of Awe, a ten-day period of introspection and repentance that culminates in Yom Kippur, also known as the Day of Atonement. These are the two holiest days of the year in the Jewish religion. Beth hoped with the new year would come new blessings and a happier and healthier year than the previous one. In a rare moment of self-reflection, as she looked back on the previous year, she felt a whirlwind of emotions. In general, she thinks she was depressed. She found herself being more short-tempered, angry, disoriented, illogical, and forgetful. She saw a change in herself that she didn't like.

Wandering around the house lost in self-reflection, Beth found herself humming. Without thinking, she found herself chanting in

Aramaic. She wasn't sure where the lyrics and melody came from, but she felt grounded. It was as if she always knew it. Stunned, she realized she was chanting the Torah portion from her bat mitzvah more than forty years earlier. She had no idea where that memory came from. But she knew it, and she was comforted by it. Finding comfort these days had been exceedingly difficult for Beth. She kept getting the feeling things weren't as they seemed or as she perceived them to be.

She even was beginning to doubt her relationship with Jim. Over the past month or two, he had been texting her and messaging her constantly, but he could never call her on the phone or video chat. There always was a crisis in his life. And he always needed her to send him money to bail him out of that problem. She would have been happy to, but he wanted her to send gift cards. She had no idea how to do that. She certainly was not going to drive to Western Union to try to figure out how to wire him money. She had no idea where there was a Western Union, anyway. It's not something that was part of her world. So she didn't send him any money, and he got angry. She grew disillusioned with him, too. She wanted more from him than texts and messages. But she didn't know how to approach it.

Besides, she had other things to worry about. The poltergeist was in rare form. She found her sneaker in the freezer next to her keys. She was tired of wiping up spills because the poltergeist moved the placemat every time she tried to put a glass or plate down. She constantly was tripping over her own feet, and in general, she was miserable. She decided to stop texting Jim. It wasn't worth it. She wasn't getting what she needed out of the relationship; she felt pressured to figure out how to send him money, felt guilty when she couldn't figure it out, and then felt frustrated she couldn't figure it out. So she stopped responding to him for a few days. He never reached out again.

She was glad for the company of the mouse. Reliably, every night he would talk to her, or more accurately, listen to her. The squirrels would chatter up a storm in her yard as they busily gathered nuts to store away for the winter. Her neighbor with the RV would come by every so often to take her places. She even made a new friend. For some reason, he never came in beyond the foyer of her house. He was tall and skinny, wore a hat and an overcoat, carried an umbrella, and never moved. But she felt him watching her as she slept, and she felt safe. She would have entire conversations with him, and he never said anything back, but he was a good listener. She decided to call him "George."

Beth still is haunted by the song "Something's Coming," but she's not convinced it's something good. She's convinced there's a huge fight going on in the world. She hears the anger in the songs in her head. She's felt fear, distrust, and anger in the world. She senses a war among the zombies and aliens and the humans. She's not sure who is allied with whom, and she's not confident about who is going to win.

Beth has started falling asleep late in the afternoon every day. That day, she woke up and it was dark out. She was entirely disoriented and afraid she was late for work. She was certain it was seven a.m. when it was seven p.m. The *West Side Story* pre-rumble song was running through her head yet again. Who was going to stop whom once and for all? Who was fighting? Was it good versus evil? Was it aliens and zombies versus humans? She decided she needed to stop watching TV. Every time she turned on the TV, there was something about an alien invasion or a zombie apocalypse and crowds of faceless people wandering the earth. People were dying everywhere. There were food shortages, natural disasters, and riots. She couldn't take it anymore.

On top of everything else, she hears bells. Every night at seven p.m. she hears what sounds like church bells ringing over and over and over again. The sound is making her crazy. There isn't a church nearby. Why does she hear bells?

She wished she could be with her family on Rosh Hashanah. But because of the danger of the zombie apocalypse, people weren't allowed to travel. She was lonely, frightened, disoriented, depressed, and angry. This wasn't the way for her to start her new year. At a visceral level, she knew she needed to clean up her act over the ten days between Rosh Hashanah and Yom Kippur. She needed to atone for her sins, apologize to anyone she may have hurt, whether on purpose or inadvertently, and she needed to pray for forgiveness. But she couldn't give herself an attitude adjustment. She was wallowing, and she knew it.

While she was entirely nonreligious, she still was culturally Jewish, and it was important to her. It felt strange to her to be alone at the High Holidays with no one but George and the mouse. At least she could livestream synagogue services over the internet and onto her TV. It made her feel less alone. This was a ceremony and prayers she had heard for more than fifty years. She recognized, remembered, and understood them. That alone gave her comfort. It grounded her a bit at a time when her reality was spinning totally out of control. She heard the ancient words, roughly translated into English as: *"May G-d bless you and protect you. May G-d smile upon you and be gracious to you. May G-d shine upon you and bless you with peace."*

And, for a few brief moments, she was at peace.

10

OCTOBER - THE TRAVEL BUG HITS

Beth's peace was short-lived. The zombies were coming out of the woodwork. While the aliens were nondescript and blended in with the neighborhoods around them, the zombies were the total opposite. They had distinct facial features, many of them with quite unkempt beards, they all looked Caucasian, and they dressed in unusual clothing. Many of them wore clothes with large letters from the alphabet on them. They favored red, white, and blue mixed with green and black camouflage. They always were in groups; it was rare to see any zombie completely alone. In the beginning of the zombie apocalypse, they were difficult to find, but as the months went by, they became more visible and vocal.

They would gather in groups in bars. They would march down the street with wooden stakes with cardboard signs on the top. The signs also had lots of large letters on them. Often, they would carry the letter Q. They would yell/shout as if to warn people they were coming. The people they came close to often turned into zombies as well. Beth found herself obsessed by letters. When she was young, she used to watch an educational TV show named *Sesame Street*. Each episode of that show was sponsored by a letter or a number, and that letter or number would be featured numerous ways throughout the TV show, for example, the letter "P" would be featured in skits about pie, or pizza, with emphasis on the letter "P." Beth couldn't figure out what the letter "Q" could be used for in a skit, other than something featuring quinoa, and that would be odd for a children's show. She was sure the zombies had to be trying to make a parody of a child's TV show. Maybe it was part of the nostalgia programming that had been showing up on numerous TV channels and in movies. Nothing else made sense. On some level, Beth was somewhat impressed with the zombies' method of recruitment/conversion. All the same, it was terrifying.

As the zombies became more and more aggressive trying to convert people into zombies, the shortage of anti-zombie products became immediately obvious. Disinfecting spray, bleach, hand sanitizer, soap and water, alcohol wipes, masks, and gloves were in noticeably short supply. People trying to avoid zombies hunkered down into their houses even more than they had before doing their best to stay away from the zombies. And yet, the zombies kept coming. They showed up in neighborhoods all over the United States, and they made their presence known.

It was as if the zombies were offended by the efficient yet quiet way the aliens were trying to protect humanity. The alien fog was subtle, and nobody knew how the aliens were able to disperse their fog so efficiently or why. The zombies denied that the aliens existed. They denied there was a fog. They denied people got well because of the fog and that the zombies were making people sick. And as more people died from the zombie attacks, the zombies grew emboldened and got louder and louder, marched more, and became angrier and angrier. The zombies bombarded social media because they couldn't get traction from traditional newscasters. And people believed them. The zombies recruited more and more people to their side, and they yelled, shouted, marched, gathered in big groups, and they posted pictures of themselves in their red hats, and they tried to take over social media. And the aliens laughed.

The aliens knew something the zombies did not. The zombies were infected, too. Every time the zombies gathered, marched, and yelled, they were infecting themselves and the aliens refused to help them with the healing fog. The zombies were killing themselves.

The scientists did their best to warn humanity about the zombies. But, protecting humanity meant humans had to change their behavior. It meant humans, normally social creatures, had to isolate from each other until the zombies killed themselves off. Most people weren't willing to do that. The scientists presented scientific evidence, and the average person listened, but others didn't. Those others became minions of the zombies and helped cleanse the planet of the pesky humans.

The wildlife was grateful. Few animals were affected by the zombies. And they started exploring through the major cities where the humans used to be. They no longer had to be afraid of the throngs of humanity around them because there weren't any. So, they wandered the planet as if they were tourists. And they liked it. There were news reports of penguins wandering the zoos visiting the polar bears. Mandarin ducks started swimming around Central Park in New York. Snowy owls flew in and out among the skyscrapers in New York and roosted in Central Park. Foxes, coyotes, and coyfoxes wandered through suburban neighborhoods, completely unafraid of the humans. Beth saw a fox and a neighborhood cat nod to each other in greeting as they each approached the trash bags left out on the street for pickup. Black bear around the country were climbing on people's decks and sunning themselves on lounge chairs. Some of the younger bears could be found splashing around in the pools in people's backyards. The animals were enjoying themselves. The humans were locked up. And Mother Nature breathed a sigh of relief that at least temporarily, humanity wasn't stressing her out, remarkably similar to the way a stay-at-home mom feels when the toddler finally goes down for a nap. There were a few hours of peace. In this case, a few months of peace. At least, it was peace on Mother Nature's part.

The scientists and medical professionals, however, were exhausted and stressed beyond all belief. They were working constantly. They would sleep in the hospital, or, if they were lucky enough to go home, they slept in their garages to protect their families from the zombies. No one was sure how long they would be able to keep working at this level of intensity without a break.

For Beth, all of this zombie tension made her feel vindicated. She had sensed something was wrong and that something was coming, something big, for months. She didn't know exactly what it was. She still wasn't exactly sure what was happening, but she could recognize something was happening that involved zombies and aliens. She had asked the mouse, the squirrels, and George, the friend who always stood by her front door, what they thought, but they didn't answer her. While she assumed her neighbors were aliens, they were so nondescript they didn't stand out as different. All of her neighbors were faceless. None of them had distinguishing features. She couldn't tell them apart. All she knew was they were kind to her.

At the same time as the zombie versus alien controversy was going on, Beth started to go stir crazy. She decided it was time to go on another business trip, even though people were told to stay at home, and she didn't have any conferences or speaking engagements booked. She began obsessing about going on an airplane with five of her close friends who also were work colleagues. She remembered vividly the layout of the plane, where people were sitting, and other details, no matter how minute. One of her friends was a six-foot-tall woman who was a patent attorney and an engineer. She had passed away a year earlier, yet Beth still saw her on that airplane.

One of her other friends was an extremely tall doctor who was nicknamed MacGyver because of his tendency to use medical tape, tongue depressors, pencil erasers, chewing gum, and whatever else he could find to create a tool when he needed something special. Clear as day, she saw the two of them busily unscrewing the seats on the airplane to give themselves more leg room. They were using random items they had either pulled from their carry-on luggage or found on the airplane and were lifting up the seats from the base of the floor to reconfigure the aircraft while the rest of the passengers were trying to get themselves on board and settled. One of her friends worked in the defense industry and was rewriting the flightpath to make it safer and more efficient. Her other friend, a therapist, was calmly trying to reassure the other passengers that Beth and her group were not going to endanger anyone. He didn't seem quite convinced himself, but he was soothing.

Beth couldn't remember when she had been on the plane with all of them, but she was certain she had been and they had another flight scheduled in the near future. She tore her desk apart trying to find the airline tickets. She went through her computer and her cell phone looking for an electronic confirmation. Even when she couldn't find a ticket, she packed her suitcase. She was sure they were all traveling together. The destination was unknown, but it was obviously a long-haul flight. Beth was researching the best airlines for lie-flat beds, the highest level of service, and the best flight schedules. One day they would be headed to Hawaii, another day to Europe, another day to Israel, another day to Australia, another day to take the Siberian railroad. While the preoccupation with the flight and details remained the same, the destination varied.

The obsession went on for weeks. She hadn't seen any of her friends in eight months because all of them were hiding in their homes to stay away from the zombies. It had been a full year since her friend was diagnosed with cancer and six months since she had passed away. Yet, the fixation about the upcoming flight continued. It was as if her mind was fighting a losing battle. The obsession about the airplane and the flight was incredibly vivid. Too vivid to be a dream, Beth thought. It had to be real. Beth could feel the hand of her seatmate lightly touch hers as they were getting settled for an extremely long flight and they jockeyed for control of the armrest. She could feel the warmth of the bowl of nuts the flight attendant handed her. Of course, they were flying first class...

She remembered puzzling why airlines would serve warm nuts with so many people who are allergic. She saw her two tall friends trying to stretch out the mattress on the lie-flat bed/seat to give themselves more room after they had MacGyvered the seats. She saw the contraption they had rigged with gum, tongue depressors, and medical tape. Not surprisingly, they seemed to have given themselves a few more inches on their seats. She heard her friends talking and laughing and could remember snippets of the conversation the next day. It was a long-haul flight with an exciting destination, clearly work-related, but also going to be fun. Beth had no idea whether it was a dream, a delusion, or reality. The world had been so strange for the past six months that she lost her ability to determine what was real and what was not.

One would assume it was a dream, but Beth didn't. The dream always was similar, exceedingly vivid, and while some of the variations were pleasant, others were terrifying, haunting Beth with feelings of being lost, being immobile, or where Beth was not able to do the things the others were able to do. In one part of the dream, for example, a van came to pick up the passengers to take them to the hotel, and Beth couldn't get into the van. She couldn't make her muscles work. She kept trying to force her legs to go up high enough to step into the van, like she was climbing a steep flight of stairs.

In another version, she and her friends were in the airport trying to get to their flight. The airport was enormous, and the moving walkways all were going in the wrong direction. After dragging their suitcases for an eternity, Beth and her friends came to a series of short zigzagging staircases. As they approached the staircases, the staircases became escalators, again going in the wrong direction. Those escalators were short, five or six steps each, didn't connect to each other in a straight line, and were separated by slippery marble flooring. They took up the center of the room as far as the eyes could see. Surrounding the escalators against the walls of the cavernous airplane terminal were mountainous staircases that looked as though they had been carved into cliffs of marble. They were terrifying. They looked as though mountain goats would have trouble climbing them. The stairs were slippery, narrow, jutting in and out from the wall at odd angles as they climbed higher, and there were no railings. It was as if someone had designed the airport terminal to mimic the most dangerous roads in the world where trucks fall off the cliff, except this design was done entirely in marble to make it even more slippery. As they climbed higher to get to their gate, Beth and her friends were joined by other random people from Beth's life. Then, one of the people fell off the cliff staircase and landed on the marble below. Obviously, she died tragically. At that point, Beth realized that not everyone traveling with them or joining them on the staircase was alive.

When she woke up, she had kicked off all the covers. Feeling relieved, Beth realized it had been a dream. As terrifying and real as it seemed, it wasn't real. At least, that's what she tried to convince herself. Her dreams, if that's what they were, left her so disoriented when she woke up that it could take her a whole day to recover. Without fail, she'd have thrown all of her bedding on the floor. If it was a particularly vivid dream, she even would have managed to dislodge the fitted sheet from the mattress as well. The first time she woke up from one of these "dreams," she was surprised to see the mouse standing outside his bureau bedroom staring at her. He was trying to figure out what all the noise had been and wanted her to shut up and go back to sleep so he could as well.

The zombie apocalypse continued. It was getting more difficult to differentiate between the currently dying and the already-had-died. And the aliens would spray entire cities with their fog, causing the inhabitants to behave like stupid, ill-behaved beasts. There were street fights and protests that verged on Civil War. Throughout the chaos, the tall, thin, nondescript people wearing navy blue sweaters stood by and watched in amazement. The zombies, seemingly unaffected by the fog, walked among the nameless, faceless humans. Newscasters got in screaming matches over whether news was real or fake. Scientists, normally revered, were accused of espousing fake news and lying to people. The world was descending into chaos. The world inside Beth's mind was even more chaotic.

Halloween was at the end of the month. Some people believe that around the time of Halloween, the veil between the living and the dead is raised and they can communicate with each other. The zombies found this whole concept amusing. After all, they were the undead, and they lived in the world between the living and the dead. They already were here. They were fascinated by the concept of children dressing up and going door to door for candy. Apparently, zombies have a sweet tooth, as do aliens. All of them thought this was one human behavior they could get behind. Then they found out that worldwide, political leaders had canceled door-to-door candy shopping, otherwise known as trick-or-treating. They were sorely disappointed.

In the meantime, Beth decided it would be a good idea for her and her colleagues to conduct business meetings in Israel and Hawaii. She has no idea why she chose those two places. So she spent hours on her computer trying to book flights. There weren't any. Furthermore, there were travel bans and the airports were closed. She thought the best idea would be to ask her neighbor with the RV if he could take them. He'd obviously had taken Beth around the world before. If he had done it once, he could do it again. Too bad she still couldn't remember his name or exactly where he lived. As frustrated as she was trying to book these flights, she was glad she had something to look forward to. She missed seeing her friends. It had been seven months since she'd seen anybody outside her neighborhood.

Beth decided she must be suffering from cabin fever. She used to get that when she was younger and growing up in New England. There were times when the snow was so bad she couldn't leave her house for a week, except on foot. She was young and impatient then, but there was always something to do. She and her sister could have fun with the neighborhood kids sledding, building snow forts and snowmen, drinking hot chocolate, and making snow ice cream. But she was with her friends and family, and it would only last a week or two. It was a novelty.

This zombie apocalypse no longer was a novelty, wasn't fun, and needed to end. Beth grew resentful of the people she saw on social media who were bored, had the time to bake bread and make cookies, start craft projects, read all of their piled-up books, and binge watch TV shows. She still had to work, even if she was working from home. It was taking her longer and longer to file her stories. Her brain wasn't working at the speed and capacity it used to. Plus, she lived alone.

There was no one to help her with any of the household chores. In the meantime, her laundry piled up, the dirty dishes piled up in the sink, she couldn't remember the last time she vacuumed or dusted, she ordered her groceries online and didn't always have time to put away the nonperishables, and she had a hard time cooking. There were days she did nothing but stare at her computer, eat or drink whatever she could find in her house, usually granola bars, chips, and protein shakes, and then she'd fall back into bed. She didn't even have time to bathe. That wasn't a huge problem. She didn't see anyone, she lived alone, and it meant she was less bothered by the shortage of shampoo and soap in the stores. There were times her online shoppers couldn't find soap or shampoo, let alone Beth's preferred brands.

She tried to control her resentment of people who had spouses or weren't working and claimed they were bored. She was quite proud that she stopped herself from yelling at her iPhone, computer, social media accounts, and the TV set. What she wanted to say was if people had so much freaking free time that they were bored with the new kinds of bread they were making, they could come to her house, do her laundry, and put it away, do her dishes, cook her some nutritious meals she just had to heat up in the microwave, put away her groceries, and edit her articles before her publishers yelled at her. She was rather impressed that she didn't say that to anyone except the mouse and the squirrels, and George, of course. At least she knew she had some discretion left. She knew she was at the end of her rope when one of her friends was complaining about not being able to throw a birthday party for a kid who was too young to even know they were having a birthday party. Instead of being able to sympathize or empathize, her thought was, "If that's the worst thing you have to worry about, get over here and do my laundry. I'm out of clean underwear!" True confession: Beth found it easier to have Alexa order her more underwear than to try to figure out how and when to do laundry. So she did. In her defense, she often would throw in a load of laundry before she started writing, get lost in her writing, forget to move the load from the washer to the dryer, and then have to rewash the load to get rid of the mildew. Even if she managed to get the laundry in both the washer and dryer, putting it away felt like an impossible task. The multicolored, morbidly obese bear on the chair was thrilled with how much laundry Beth fed him. He especially appreciated that the laundry always was clean. Ordering more underwear was an easy option for Beth. She had to yell at Alexa while she was doing something else, and Alexa would take care of it.

Speaking of Alexa, Beth was growing more frustrated with the technology around her house. Siri and Alexa had some gripe with each other. Alexa was in charge of the music, the lights, and shopping. Siri was in charge of the calendar, the weather reports, and the reminders. Siri spent a lot of time talking to herself. She'd hear something on TV, her voice would come out of the telephone, and the iPad would answer. The iPhone and the iPad could continue their discussion for hours. It would stop if Beth overheard and told Siri to stop talking. Alexa was becoming quite bossy. She would make helpful suggestions at random times throughout the day such as, "Would you like to hear a joke?" Or, "Why don't you ask me, Alexa where's my stuff?" It was as if she was eavesdropping. Beth got used to hearing, "Sorry, I don't have an answer for that," when she hadn't asked anything. It didn't matter whether Beth was in the same room as Siri or Alexa, the disembodied voices answered unspoken questions no matter where she was.

Even more annoying, however, were the incessant requests for passwords from her phone, iPad, and laptop. Beth would be in the middle of doing something, and the phone would decide it needed to lock and she needed to type in a password to restart it. The iPad would do the same thing. The computer, not to be upstaged, would pick the most inopportune times to do updates and then demand a computer restart before it would work properly again. It was like it was going on strike, or at least threatening to. Every time Beth had to stop what she was doing to key in a password, she would forget what she was doing before she had to key in the password. It kept getting worse as she got worse about remembering her passwords. She was beginning to feel like her life was being ruled by technology instead of the technology assisting her.

Beth knew the world was broken. It was clear that between the zombies and technology taking over the world, the world was doomed. Most days, she felt like she was the only one who saw it. She got the feeling other people couldn't see what she saw, that the world was being dismantled person by person and piece by piece. If the poltergeists had replaced her real items with counterfeit ones, it stood to reason that other poltergeists were doing the same thing throughout the planet. She could see the zombies for what they were. Why couldn't everyone else? Perhaps her sense of déjà vu was a psychic strength brought on by her collection of sea glass and moon stones. She found that thought mildly humorous. She'd be the first psychic superhero who tripped over her own feet and dropped things all the time.

11

NOVEMBER - THANKSGIVING

Beth could not believe how quickly time flew by. One day it was Rosh Hashanah, and it seemed like the next day was Thanksgiving. The zombies were completely out of control. They were taking over airports, clogging up highways, and invading the homes of their family members and friends. The zombies were doing their best to convert people to their side.

It was at this time the mouse asked Beth if he could bring over some friends. He said he was afraid for them to continue living outside with everything going on. "Of course, you can," Beth replied, "this is your house, too. And if you're afraid for them, they probably should plan to move in and stay here until it becomes safe again. We have plenty of space." Naturally, Beth assumed the mouse was talking about other mice. Much to her surprise, the mouse ran into the kitchen, walked under the doorway into the laundry room, and disappeared behind the water heater.

"Be right back," he called over his shoulder. A few minutes later, the mouse popped out from behind the water heater with a trail of diminutive people carrying luggage. They looked like average people, except they were the size of a mouse, and were purple. There were at least two dozen purple people, dressed in wildly colorful clothing with mismatched patterns, carrying a variety of objects. Some were pushing wheelbarrows filled with pots and pans and camp stoves, some were carrying suitcases, some had the fancy four-wheeled suitcases Beth had always admired, still others had what looked like pet carriers, and everyone had backpacks. While they were colorful, cheerful, and incredibly grateful to Beth for letting them in, she couldn't help but think they looked like refugees. She had the impression they literally were carrying everything they owned with them. She half-expected to see a covered wagon following them. As they walked through the kitchen and into the dining room, some people in the group spotted the boy and girl statues. As always, the girl was holding a bowl of candy, and the boy was holding a bottle of lime. They stopped in their tracks, turned as one to face the boy and girl, smiled, and bowed down before them.

Much to Beth's surprise, the boy and girl became animated and made motions for the diminutive people to stand up and stop bowing. "You are welcome here, and you're safe," they said, echoing the words Beth had spoken to them earlier. And then, the boy and girl shrunk down to be the size of the diminutive people and led them into the sunroom. There, they introduced them to the fox who smiled widely as he said hello. At first, they were frightened because when he smiled, they could see his teeth, and they knew foxes usually eat mice. They were afraid the fox might be looking at them as a meal because they were mouse size. But the fox set their minds at ease and said he viewed them as roommates and not as dinner. The mouse and the boy and girl assured them this was the case, and they were safe.

Beth was wondering what shelter they would like to live in. They were so small and scared. Then she realized they weren't afraid of her; they were afraid of the zombies. They introduced themselves individually, and Beth hoped she could remember their names. The mouse motioned to her to follow him, and they went into the bedroom.

"Don't worry about remembering their names," he said. "They can't remember their own names." He explained further, "They all have their given names which is what they told you. Then, they all have their nicknames which they use with each other. And then, the parents use different names for the children. I've found they'll answer to pretty much anything." He continued, "Watch the first time one of the mothers needs to reprimand one of her children. She'll run through a list of five or six names and then say something like 'You know which one of you I mean!' and they will know."

Beth smiled, because she had many friends who when faced with that situation would run through all of the names of all of their children, the dog, and the cat to try to remember the name of the one they were trying to reprimand. Apparently, this was a cross-cultural phenomenon.

Beth and the mouse went back into the sunroom where the fox was engaged in earnest conversation with the diminutive people. He explained he would keep to his den under the coffee table, and he most certainly would not encroach on any space they wanted to use in the sunroom. He highly recommended the sunroom. He said it was his favorite room in the house other than the kitchen and the garage where there was food, but it was too cold to sleep in the garage and Beth wouldn't let them sleep in the kitchen. The mouse pointed out that he slept under the bureau in Beth's bedroom. He suggested at first that they might want to live under the sofa in the sunroom, but then he quickly recognized they might be too vulnerable. The sofa backed up to the sliding glass doors in the sunroom, and the back of the sofa was visible to the street unless the blinds were totally closed. It was a catch-22 because if the blinds were totally closed, the sunroom wasn't as sunny and got cold, but with them open getting the sun, the diminutive people could be seen from the street.

The boy and the girl grew back to their original size, told the diminutive people to wait for a minute, and they went exploring through the house. They came back with two suggestions: First, they wondered if living under the king-sized bed in the guest bedroom was a good option, or would the diminutive people prefer to build their own village out of the assorted-sized Amazon boxes Beth had been keeping in the garage once she emptied them of her deliveries? The boy and the girl took a blanket from the sofa and spread it out on the floor so everyone could have a comfortable place to sit. The discussion became quite lively as the diminutive people realized they had multiple good options, they were safe, they were warm, and the zombies couldn't get them inside Beth's house. Even as they had this discussion, the fox's hackles rose. He could see the zombies looking through the mist surrounding Beth's house and trying to peek through the windows to see who or what was inside. But for some reason, even though everyone inside could see out and could come and go as they pleased, the zombies were repelled. It was as if Beth's house was zombie-proof.

It scared the diminutive people, though, enough that they chose to move out of the sunroom and build their village under the king-sized bed in the guestroom. Beth thought the location was good, but she felt badly that they were sleeping on a hardwood floor. After all, the mouse had built himself a nest, and the fox had built a den lined with blankets. All she could think of was the extra bathmat from the guest bathroom, or some towels or blankets. All of her roommates, old and new, thought the bathmat was a great idea, particularly since it was memory foam and oversized. Ever the good host, Beth went to the guest bathroom, grabbed the bathmat, and put it under the bed. As she returned to the conversation in the sunroom, the discussion stopped abruptly as the participants, including the fox and the mouse, looked behind Beth with their mouths agape. There, walking from the dining room through the living room was Einstein and the Mad Hatter. They were about four inches high and were stretching as they walked. It was like they were shaking tension out of their arms, shoulders, and legs.

"We've been living on the side of the refrigerator for a year," Einstein explained. "We were afraid to let anyone know we were alive, so we pretended to be refrigerator magnets. But we know it's safe, and we are sore!" Addressing the diminutive people, the Mad Hatter asked if it was okay if he and Einstein joined them in their new home under the bed.

The fox, the mouse, and the boy and the girl were staring at each other in disbelief. They could not believe that none of them had recognized that the Mad Hatter and Einstein were alive. But then Einstein pointed out they had purposely tried to hide, and none of the others should blame themselves.

On some level, the Mad Hatter and the diminutive people had the same fashion sense. While Einstein wore a navy-blue suit, the Mad Hatter had a green jacket, checkerboard pants, a red tie, and a black hat. He fit right in. Einstein was, well, Einstein. He was welcome anywhere. So, the diminutive people accompanied by Einstein and the Mad Hatter moved into their new home under the guest bed and began to unpack. Beth wanted to make sure they had something to eat, a bathroom, a shower, running water, and other things she assumed they needed. But, she had to admit she was completely unaware of what they truly would want or need. So she asked them.

It turns out they did have pets in the pet carriers. They asked if she had any dog food or dog treats. Of course she did. She took a small dessert plate from the kitchen and filled it with assorted dog treats and pieces of dog kibble. The diminutive people were amazed. They also found it humorous. Clearly, Beth had no idea how much food she had given them. One dog cookie could feed all of their pets for two weeks. Beth had given them about a year's worth of food. The mouse said he'd be happy to eat some of that, and the fox did, too. Beth told him there was plenty more, so they should enjoy themselves. The fox smiled at Beth and told her that he had already learned to open the cabinet and help himself. He would take responsibility for feeding the diminutive dogs.

That left food for the people, water, and bathrooms/showers. It turned out the people were scavengers and had been forced to eat whatever they could find. Recently, because it was winter, they had depended on birdseed, and trash people had left in the street. They were too short to climb into the garbage cans or dumpsters. The fox was heartbroken. He himself was an expert scavenger and quite adept at knocking garbage cans over so he could get out the contents. He didn't realize the diminutive people were following behind him and eating whatever was left on the ground. He apologized, but they said it wasn't necessary. Without him, they would've lost all access to the trash cans and the food inside.

Moving forward, Beth told them they did not need to eat trash and leftovers anymore, like the fox and the mouse didn't. She asked the diminutive people what they enjoyed eating. It turns out the diminutive people were junk food junkies. Their idea of health-food was canned fruit, the stickier the better, and their favorite foods were cookies, crackers, and cheese. Beth had tons available. They pointed out to her that one can of fruit was enough to feed their entire village for a week, and they would be thrilled.

And then one of the youngest piped up, "Do you have any chocolate?" The whole village laughed. They each had sweet a tooth, but as the saying goes, "Out of the mouths of babes." No adult had the guts to ask for candy. Beth had an entire bag of assorted candy stashed from Halloween. It would be enough to feed the village for years, even after she gorged herself. So, she went into the kitchen and made a plate for the village. She gave them a cheese stick, an open can of fruit, and two miniature candy bars. They were thrilled, obviously. But she still hadn't figured out beverages and bathrooms. So, she asked. The mouse handled that question. He showed them the tiny hole in the wall behind the water heater leading outside to where he had built a full, mouse-sized bathroom. He had taken insulation from Beth's garage to insulate it. He also had made a shower, a sink, and multiple toilet stalls. Since he had moved in with Beth, he no longer needed to use his energy searching for food or shelter, so he indulged his carpentry skills. He told them they were totally welcome to use the outdoor bathroom anytime they wanted. Beth realized she had been living twelve feet away from a construction site for a year, and never heard the mouse and his building. She was impressed he was so quiet. Some of the human builders could use a lesson from him.

Einstein and the Mad Hatter were thrilled with their new food and shelter options, and they welcomed the company. They, however, were too large to fit through the mouse hole to get to the outdoor bathroom. Einstein, clearly a genius, pointed out they could use the en suite bathroom attached to the guest room. They were bigger than the diminutive people, and that made Beth's bathroom a viable option for them. They admitted they would not be able to lift or put down the toilet seat, nor would they be able to flush. The fox said he would take care of it. The boy and the girl smiled, because they also knew they could take care of it as well. Throughout all of these conversations, George, the man who always stood by the door, remained silent. He didn't participate at all.

In the meantime, Beth was amazed at the village being built under her guest bed. She had grown up reading *Gulliver's Travels* and *Horton Hears a Who* but had thought those were works of fiction. Clearly, Beth thought, she had been mistaken because obviously they were real. They were right there in front of her and under her bed. They had built an entire town under there. With her permission, the boy and the girl had moved some of the plant pots that now housed dormant bulbs from the sunroom to under the bed. The villagers used the pots and the dead leaves.

They built their communal buildings at the top of each branch of the plant, connected by long slides constructed of leaves. The houses were raised up from the soil. Directly on the soil were miniature grocery stores, shops, a school, and the library. They had chosen three pots with one amaryllis bulb in each. The plants had never flowered and never grew more than two leaves per plant. There was a lot of space in the pots. Beth was impressed at their ingenuity. The plant pots were under the bed next to the bathmat. The bathmat was lined with multiple sleeping bags, pillows, blankets, and dog beds. The plates of food were on the bathmat, as well. Beth was amazed at the tenacity of the diminutive people. They built quickly, and happily settled in.

So after that night, Beth's little household grew. She was living with her roommates: George, the mouse, the fox, the boy, the girl, Einstein, the Mad Hatter, and an entire village of diminutive people. She was happy, and honestly, if she admitted it to herself, she felt safer with everyone around.

The zombie apocalypse was in full force at Thanksgiving. People had been hiding in their houses for six months and were completely unaware the zombie apocalypse was growing exponentially and what they should have been afraid of. Beth knew something that other people didn't. She knew many people were imposters. They looked like familiar people. They acted like familiar people, but Beth knew they were imposters and were zombies. Beth knew the zombies took advantage of the fact that people saw what they wanted to see so the people would believe it was their loved one when really it was a zombie. The zombies were efficiently infecting people one at a time, and it was always the people closest to the uninfected. The zombies took advantage of peoples' anxiety, depression, and loneliness and gathered their loved ones together for Thanksgiving; thereby infecting them much more effectively and efficiently and converting those people to zombies, too. And people died. And the zombies denied it. The zombies had to deny it, quite frankly. Because, if they had admitted they were spreading death, they would lose all credibility, and no one would want to be around them. Then, they could not convert people to their side. So, the zombies denied any problem, pretended nothing was wrong, and continued to do whatever they wanted. And people let them.

Beth missed her family, too. But she had always trusted science and science was saying to stay away from people, so she stayed away from the people she loved. Even so, the isolation was getting to her. Beth got angry. While one could justify much of her anger, many times it was unprovoked anger, a complete overreaction, and out of the blue. She started scaring herself.

In some ways, her anger was reasonable. She wanted to see family and friends, go shopping, go to a restaurant, fly back to Florida to see her parents, pick her own groceries instead of having them delivered, get a haircut, get her nails and eyebrows done, and other things that gave her pleasure and helped her relax. But she didn't because she didn't want to help the zombies convert people, and she didn't want to expose anyone else or be exposed to the zombie plague. Again, her frustration and anger was, on some level, reasonable. On the other hand, things she used to find mildly annoying or even funny were making her blow her top. She got miffed at her computer, iPhone, and iPad. Some might say that was a reasonable reaction because it was as if the computer's sole goal in life was to make her life more difficult. Clearly, the iPhone and the iPad were her computer's allies.

For example, she wanted to ship chocolate-covered caramel apples to friends and family. She tried to do so on her iPhone, and the website wouldn't work. She tried to do so on her iPad, and the website wouldn't work. She went to her computer which decided now was the time to do extensive updates, and it needed to restart. Every time she tried to delay the updates, another pop-up blocked her screen and told her updates were needed. That, of course, happened after her computer had turned itself off and restarted and needed her to login again. It lost her place on the website. As a matter of fact, it completely closed the website, and Beth couldn't remember the name of the store. She had tried to avoid this situation by leaving the browser open to the website she wanted to order from.

She finally got the website open, carefully chose the apples she wanted to send, went to another site to order gift bags and tissue paper, and congratulated herself on the spectacular plan of having all the apples delivered to her so she could put them in the gift bags with tissue paper and deposit them on the doorsteps of her friends and neighbors like a Jewish elf. The frustration of using three electronic devices was superseded by her joy at choosing which person would like which apple in the anticipation of walking through her neighborhood, stealthily leaving presents at people's doors. Until she tried to place the orders, however. Her $200 order for apples was going to cost her $700 to ship and probably wouldn't be delivered until after Christmas. Arriving after Christmas wasn't a huge problem, particularly since these were not Christmas gifts, but the $700 was a big problem. She tried to find an alternative, but quickly gave up. That was a good thing. It turns out the gift bags and the tissue paper wouldn't arrive until mid-January. "Sorry, everyone. You're not getting a holiday surprise from me this year," she thought.

She was her "normal" self during this process: mildly aggravated and frustrated, but totally able to see the humor in spending $700 to ship apples. The ridiculousness of it made her grin and start looking for alternative chocolate caramel apples. Then she thought about other foods or small gifts she could give. The purpose wasn't to give an exotic expensive gift, it was to bring joy to her friends and neighbors who were shut in because of the zombie infestation/alien invasion. Let's not forget it was flu season as well. Still, neither the flu nor zombies justified $700 shipping. She found herself smiling at the absurdity when she added up the cost of the apples, the shipping, gift bags, tissue paper, and the rush shipping to get the gift bags and tissue paper before the middle of January, it was going to cost her over one thousand dollars. That would mean her little holiday pick-me-up gift would cost roughly $75 per person. We all know that a $75 apple is an awfully expensive piece of fruit. She found it funny. Clearly this was not going to happen. The technology deserved to die, however, in her humble opinion.

While she could laugh off the $75 apples, she completely blew up, every pun intended, when she opened a case of soda and one of the cans inside was completely bulging at the top to the point she couldn't lift the metal tab. She yelled at the can while trying to figure out how to either open the soda and pour the contents down the sink or throw out the can of soda without having it explode all over the trashcan. She figured something was wrong with it so drinking it was not a particularly good idea. She had eleven other cans in the case, so it was not a huge problem to not drink this one can of soda. And, as we discussed earlier, she had enough cases of soda to build a wall in the garage. Yet, this one can of soda made her lose it.

After ranting at the soda for more than half an hour, trying to lift the tab with her hand, trying to use the little device she got to help open hard-to-open tabs without breaking a fingernail, trying to pry it open with a knife, and a few other equally as ineffective ways to open the can, she gave up. Giving up completely, however, was not an option. She was far too angry. So, it still sits on the counter mocking her a week later. Once she calmed down, Beth was a bit taken aback by the level of rage she had felt at the can of soda. There was no need for it, but she couldn't control herself. It was a complete white-hot rage that welled up inside her from nowhere. Fortunately, the target of the rage was a can of soda, not another person. But it was out of character for her. Normally, her anger didn't get to quite that level, her anger was usually provoked by something she sees as unfair or unjust, particularly if it hurts another person she cares about, but this was entirely different. It came out of nowhere.

The can of soda was still on the counter when Beth decided to revisit the gift challenge. Refusing to go into a store during a zombie apocalypse for gifts for other people when she was having everything she needed for herself delivered so she could stay safe seemed like the most logical choice. Besides, she was an expert online shopper and quite adept at getting things shipped to her, the $700 apples notwithstanding. So she checked out three bakeries, four candy shops, and a gourmet food store from Boston under the assumption something that had good memories for her would be something her friends and neighbors would enjoy. Not a single one of them could guarantee delivery in the month of December. This was a new phenomenon for her, by the way. Beth, as we mentioned, doesn't celebrate Christmas. Usually, she would run to a gourmet store and pick up a few little tchotchkes here and there so she would have gifts for hostess gifts or in case someone dropped by and brought something for her.

All of her friends knew that day-after-Christmas-sale was her favorite holiday. People might get gifts for random reasons, just because they were on sale. But she never had any Christmas time pressure for shopping. In her world, she would send gifts to people's kids, have small gifts to give out at her holiday party, but had never experienced $700 to ship an apple, gifts not arriving by Christmas, or anything like that. After checking with a bunch of friends, she found out that apparently, she could not blame the zombies for this. Her friends who do celebrate Christmas told her that Black Friday shopping is a great idea except you have to be able to hand the gifts to people because you often need more time to wrap and ship than you would expect. That was the end of the holiday gift-giving fiasco for the year. Over and done.

It was around this time the work-related virtual meetings escalated to the point of ridiculousness. At one point, she had regular phone calls coming in on her cell phone, a FaceTime call coming in on her iPad, a WhatsApp call ringing, and a calendar reminder popping up about the Microsoft teams call starting in one minute, all while she was on a Zoom call. That didn't include the texts and emails coming in at the same time.

Beth was exhausted. There's no other way around it. She had to work harder and harder to complete anything. Part of the problem definitely was the constant interruptions while she was trying to write. But there was a part of her wondering why those interruptions were disturbing her. She used to be able to concentrate and ignore the messages popping up on the computer screen, or the dinging of the texts, or the ringing of the phone. Everything was a distraction, even the cars driving by on the street. Yet, as exhausted as she was, every night she would try to fall asleep and couldn't. She felt like she was being watched. From her bedroom, she could see that the fox had moved into the sunroom and slept under the coffee table. It was brightly colored: it was orange, had a bright fuchsia tail, and wore blue socks. It was friendly looking. It didn't make sense to her why the fox was in her sunroom, nor did it make sense why it would wear socks, but she felt like it was watching out for her.

The mouse would still come in every night to say goodnight before sleeping under the bureau. It was puzzling as to why the fox did not eat the mouse, but since they seemed to get along, she decided not to worry about it. George, the friend who stood by her front door, still wearing his hat and coat and carrying his umbrella, had no advice about this either.

Not wanting to seem inhospitable but curious just the same, Beth decided to address the fox directly. She said the fox was welcome to stay in the sunroom, but she was curious as to why it chose to do so. The fox replied that it had lived in the neighborhood for years. It made a habit of visiting people, usually by sitting on their balconies or patios, making friends with their pets, and in general, hanging out. It also enjoyed going through people's trash since it saved the fox lots of time and energy instead of hunting. The fox continued, "Your house came highly recommended by the squirrel family. They said you were nice, your house was quite comfortable, and you are always pleased to feed them their favorite foods. Then I talked to the mouse. The mouse said he comes over to your house every night and sleeps under your bureau. It's getting cold out, and people are acting strangely, so I figured I'd stay here, too. I hope it's not a problem!"

Beth still was concerned about whether the fox would eat the mouse or the squirrels, but she hesitated in bringing it up. The fox must have anticipated her question. He told her that he and the other wildlife in her neighborhood had struck an agreement. Since the food supply was so plentiful with the plants, the dumpster behind the restaurants, and people's trash, they no longer needed to be predator and prey. Instead, they considered each other neighbors.

Making sure she understood, Beth clarified, "So you are not going to eat or hunt or hurt the mouse or the squirrels, right?" The fox agreed.

Mollified, Beth told the fox he was welcome to stay and carried him to the kitchen. She asked what his favorite foods were so she could show him what she had. The fox was excited about her frozen mixed berries, the nut and seed mix the squirrels also liked, her salad mix, and then was ecstatic when he discovered the cabinet containing the dog treats. He was particularly thrilled by the single-ingredient dog treats that were chicken, beef, or fish. Then, she showed him the other freezer, the one in the garage, and his eyes lit up. He was excited to try the uncooked chicken, the frozen turkey, and the hamburger.

"I'll find plenty to eat!" he exclaimed.

Satisfied she could take care of the fox safely, Beth was happy to have him as an unofficial roommate. She asked where he wanted to sleep. He said he enjoyed the area under the coffee table in the sunroom because it was like a den with a good view. He did ask if he could take the blanket off of the sofa, though. Beth happily complied.

She arranged it under the table, and gently laid the fox down on it. He looked totally content. She wondered if the fox was housebroken. Just in case, she put out some dog peepee pads and told the fox she didn't want to insult him, that he was more than welcome to go outside or use the toilet, but that the peepee pads were there if he needed them. He grinned at her and gave a wag of his tail.

While she was giving the fox a tour of the kitchen, boy and girl sculptures walked into the kitchen and introduced themselves to the fox. He answered back. The girl offered the fox candy from her bowl. The boy did not offer the fox any wine, by the way. Beth asked the boy and the girl when they became able to walk. They smiled at her, winked at the fox, and said to her, "We'll never tell!" And they happily trotted around the house playing. They were roughly the height of three-year-olds, dressed in brightly colored clothes, and the fox wiggled to get down and play with them. They had a blast chasing each other around. George watched over them silently. The mouse watched from a distance. He clearly was afraid he could get run over.

Saying goodnight to the fox, George, the children, the residents of plant-land, and the mouse, Beth turned off the light, snuggled under the covers, and tried to fall asleep. As she dozed off, Beth saw pictures of horses and carriages floating through her mind. Some looked like Cinderella's carriage, others looked like the horse and buggies that would go through Central Park, and still others looked like the pumpkin being pulled by mice. It was as if every children's book had been rolled into one and the combinations of horses, carriages, mice, pumpkins, fairy godmothers, clocks, and everything else had been combined with the magic carpet ride. She couldn't make sense of it.

Soon after she dozed off, there was a knock at her door. Looking at her smart phone, she realized it was only seven p.m. She hadn't realized how early it was when she thought it was time to go to bed. Fortunately, she still had all of her clothes on. She answered the door and was pleased to see her neighbor with the RV. She was embarrassed that she couldn't recognize his face or remember his name, but she knew she felt safe with him, so that was enough. He asked her if she might be interested in going on a road trip. She didn't want to be rude to George, the friend who always stood by the door, so she asked her neighbor if he could come, too. The neighbor looked at her oddly and said he was more than welcome to come some other time, but this time, Beth should come by herself. George, still standing motionless and silent by the door, didn't object.

Beth put on her shoes, grabbed her coat and gloves, and followed her neighbor out the front door. This time, she remembered her phone, pocketbook, and keys. She was rather pleased with herself. This time, there were a few of her neighbors in the RV. They all wore camel-hair overcoats over their navy-blue sweaters, and Beth was embarrassed that to her, they all looked completely indistinguishable. There were no differentiating facial features, no variation in their clothes, nothing that could help her tell them apart. They all greeted her warmly and offered her the seat of honor, the front passenger seat. There was an animated discussion behind her among her neighbors. The debate was whether or not one needed mini marshmallows, large marshmallows, or no marshmallows in the hot chocolate. Beth smiled to herself. Obviously, the answer was mini marshmallows. If one wants to be extremely picky about it, dehydrated mini marshmallows are the best in hot chocolate, she thought. They don't get nearly as sticky as the other ones.

The RV flew just above Route I-95 and the New Jersey Turnpike. In a few minutes, barely enough time for the water to boil for the hot chocolate, they were in New York City. The neighbors finished making the hot chocolate and gave each person their own thermos. Beth was curious to see the result of the marshmallow debate while, at the same time, she didn't want to seem overeager and open hers immediately. Miracle of miracles, the neighbor driving the RV found a parking space on the street a few steps away from the Plaza Hotel. And there, across the street from the RV, stood horses and buggies of every sort one could imagine. There even was a small pumpkin surrounded by some mice. All that was missing was the fairy godmother and a magic carpet. Beth was both thrilled and amazed.

Reaching into the luggage compartment under the RV, Beth's neighbor pulled out a suitcase. It had Beth's name on it. "We took the liberty of packing for you," he said. "We thought you could use a break. You've been stressed recently." And there, standing on the steps of the Plaza

Hotel, were Beth's friends. Her work/travel companions, her sister, and her parents were smiling and waving. They didn't seem even remotely surprised to see her. Obviously, all of them were in on the surprise.

"Don't worry," said Beth's neighbor. "We'll protect all of you from the zombies. You can be close together, hug, eat, talk, walk anywhere you want to, and for a day or two, you can behave like you were before the zombie apocalypse." Then, a bubble enveloped Beth and the rest of her group. It moved with them, and everyone in that bubble was safe. This was the first time in six months that any of them had hugged each other.

Beth and her group walked into the hotel, and the bellhop took them to their rooms. A few minutes later, they gathered in the one restaurant that was open in the hotel... it happened to be one of Beth's favorites. As they sat at their table in the Palm Court, the waitstaff brought over an incredible tray of goodies and a bottle of champagne. The tea service had something for everyone: tea, caviar, savory sandwiches, petite sweets, and upscale bar food like lobster rolls and gourmet hamburger sliders. It was spectacular. The food was great, the atmosphere was wonderful, and the company was even better. Beth had been yearning for that normalcy for months.

Later that evening, everyone bundled up to take a horse and carriage ride around Central Park. It turned out everyone had been given a thermos of hot chocolate by her neighbors, and it still was hot. Beth wondered where her neighbors had bought the thermoses. They were excellent at keeping things hot for quite a long time. Beth and her "entourage" went to the largest carriage they saw, and it was, indeed, large enough to accommodate all of them. There was one problem, however, Beth couldn't get into the carriage. The driver had put a stepstool up to help her, and she couldn't make her leg lift up to get on the stepstool or to get up the step to the carriage. She didn't know why, because she was significantly taller than some of the other people who hopped up with no problem. But she couldn't make herself do it. She was getting frustrated, embarrassed, and angry; she was literally stuck standing there unable to make her body do what she wanted and needed it to do. And then her neighbor appeared at her side and one of her friends appeared at her other side.

The friend looked deep into her eyes and said, "We will get you up here. You're safe, and you don't need to worry." Beth calmed down and stopped struggling. Her leg still wouldn't work, and her arm and hand had lost their strength so she couldn't pull herself up, but she knew it was going to be okay. Her friend and her neighbor stood shoulder to shoulder with her and she became stronger. She climbed up into the carriage with no problem. She'd gotten used to tripping over her own feet, dropping things, and not having the strength she used to, but she never had experienced anything quite like this. She was glad her friend and neighbor were there to help her and no one else made a big deal about it. She was embarrassed. Even more than that, she was scared. Something was wrong.

She almost immediately forgot about the "incident," however. It was so wonderful to be with the people closest to her, to snuggle under blankets that protected them against the cold, to drink hot chocolate (with dehydrated marshmallows, by the way), and to enjoy the sights of Manhattan. There weren't many people to watch, and those they did see were entirely faceless. Their clothing was incredibly high fashion, however. Beth enjoyed looking at that. She was amazed people in Manhattan could make winter coats, boots, hats, and gloves look beautiful. She no longer was surprised people didn't have faces. She realized that even the people in her group, whom she'd known for years, even decades, didn't have faces either. But, she knew who they were, so she didn't worry. It was interesting how faceless people were becoming normal.

The rest of the minivacation at the hotel was almost normal. At least, it was as normal as it could be with most restaurants closed, the spas closed, and Broadway closed. But Beth and her family and friends were able to relax, enjoy great food and company, and genuinely appreciate luxury accommodations. In some ways, it was nicer than normal. The hotel wasn't crowded, they didn't have to push and shove their way down streets in New York, and they got to talk to each other. There was far less tumult than usual.

When the weekend was over, Beth rode home in the RV with her neighbors. She wasn't sure how her family and friends got home, and she forgot to worry about it until she got home. She never found out the answer. She was relaxed and eternally grateful when she returned home. She hadn't realized how completely stressed she had been until the stress was gone. For the first time in a long time, she felt clear-headed and energized.

She was thrilled she had gotten to see people she cared about in person. When Thanksgiving rolled around, she was even happier she had been able to see people "in real life," as they say.

This was the year of the Zoom and FaceTime Thanksgiving. Families would get together in their own houses and video call each other so they could spend the holidays "together" without endangering anybody's health. It felt strange for Beth not to be hosting her traditional "Friendsgiving" dinner on the Saturday after Thanksgiving. That was a time for friends and family to gather together in a relaxed atmosphere after spending traditional Thanksgiving with their family. The rules of Friendsgiving were simple: If you missed your favorite Thanksgiving dish because you went to somebody else's house and they didn't serve it, you needed to cook it or buy it and bring it, making sure to bring enough for others to share; dress in your comfortable clothes; and be prepared for a buffet-style dinner. The most important rule, however, was you had to bring your own containers for leftovers. There always were plenty of leftovers, but containers have a way of disappearing into other people's houses and never coming back. It gets expensive to have to keep buying brand-new plastic containers. This year, however, the 22-pound turkey sitting in Beth's chest freezer in the garage never saw the light of day. It will stay there until, well, whenever.

The Zoom Friendsgiving call was fun, even though it was different. People were eating all sorts of food, most of it completely unrelated to Thanksgiving, and pretty much what they normally would have brought to Beth's house. People of different ethnicities have different traditions. Few of Beth's friends craved the traditional American Thanksgiving meal of turkey, stuffing/dressing, mashed potatoes, green bean casserole, macaroni and cheese, white dinner rolls, and pie. Instead, the Friendsgiving dinners were representative of the diversity of her friends' backgrounds and included Jewish food like kasha and bowties, knishes, kugel, and often a brisket; Chinese food like stir-fried dry tofu, Dungeness crab, fish, and assorted noodle dishes; Filipino food like lumpia; Korean food like seafood pancakes; Italian food like ravioli and burrata; and Polish food like stuffed cabbage and pierogi.

All cultures agreed on the necessity of pie, however. There were many years when there was one pie per person resulting from the scavenger hunt Beth and her friends embarked on while searching for the best pie. That scavenger hunt took them to some unusual places. Unfortunately, the best pie was a four-hour round-trip, and the bakery recently went out of business. Beth and her friends had stored unbaked frozen pies from that bakery for months, but by now they were long gone. The temptation was too much, and the pies were devoured. The annual pre-Thanksgiving pie scavenger hunt and face-to-face Friendsgiving were traditions everyone missed. A Zoom holiday couldn't replace it. But it was better than nothing.

While Beth was unhappy about not having Thanksgiving or Friendsgiving at her house, she was a bit relieved. She'd been having an extremely difficult time cooking. She was leaving ingredients out of recipes she'd made for decades. She was having a much harder time remembering what ingredients she needed to buy in order to bake. She used to be able to have multiple dishes in various stages of preparation all going on at the same time. For example, if she had three recipes involving chopped apples with cinnamon and sugar, she would chop all of the apples she needed for the recipes, put them in a big bowl, and use them as she needed. She couldn't do that anymore. It struck her as odd, but she also realized she hated cooking just for herself. She was much happier cooking for a room full of people. She decided she was messing up the recipes because she didn't care enough. Or, at least that's what she was trying to convince herself.

12

DECEMBER - THE DESCENT

December started out oddly. Beth was scared. She couldn't shake this feeling that something terrible was happening. She couldn't tell exactly what was wrong; all she knew was something was very, very wrong. She constantly felt like someone was watching her. It wasn't the comforting "watching out for her" she experienced with her neighbors, George, the squirrels, the fox, and the mouse. Instead, she felt like somebody was watching her. She found herself spending more time each day making sure all of the windows and the doors were locked. She constantly was on edge and angry at the poltergeist. The poltergeist stole things as well as moving them. Her pocketbook went missing. Her cell phone went missing. The money she knew she had in her bureau drawer went missing. The poltergeist was clearly changing the passwords on her computer on a regular basis. She kept getting locked out of her laptop and iPad. Beth felt she was living this day over and over again. She'd go to sleep, wake up, live the same day, and repeat. It was like a horrible version of Groundhog Day.

In addition to the overwhelming feeling of déjà vu, Beth noticed other bizarre things happening. She woke up one morning and smelled...

Nothing. She noticed the absence of smell because things she normally could and would smell just weren't there. For example, she had an old heating system and it always smelled hot. It's hard to describe, but the heat had a definite smell to it. Plus, the windows in the house were old, and Beth could always smell the fresh air from the outside, which was good, and the exhaust fumes from the trucks and the snowplows going by, which was bad.

Today, she smelled nothing. It became even more obvious something was wrong when she microwaved a packet of oatmeal and smelled nothing. She double checked the label, and it said it was cinnamon and spice. She decided it was a cheap brand of instant oatmeal, so she added in a handful of raisins and extra cinnamon hoping to improve on it. She stirred the oatmeal, she still smelled nothing. She let it sit to cool off and thicken before she took a bite. It is difficult to describe what Beth felt when she put it in her mouth. She could feel the raisins against her tongue, she could feel the spice tingling on her tongue, but she couldn't smell or taste anything. Cursing herself for buying the cheapest oatmeal she could find instead of her usual, favorite brand, she decided that not all generics were the same. But since she had already made the oatmeal, she decided to eat it anyway. It didn't smell or taste like anything, but at least it made her feel full.

Later that morning, Beth realized she had forgotten to drink a protein shake. Being a transplanted Bostonian, the cold, snowy weather outside was not a deterrent to Beth's drinking iced coffee instead of hot. She took the pot of iced coffee out of the refrigerator, put it in her blender, and added a coffee protein shake. She blended the shake, took off the blade attachment to put on the drinking attachment, and realized the coffee didn't smell. She understood the coffee protein shake didn't smell that strongly because it never did. But, even iced coffee usually smells like coffee, although admittedly, less like coffee than hot coffee does. Sighing to herself, Beth entertained the thought that she might have yet another sinus infection. It was funny, though, her nose didn't feel particularly stuffy. She drank the iced coffee, not able to smell it, and not tasting anything, but not particularly concerned since she assumed she had a sinus infection.

Beth decided to take some decongestant, some antihistamine, and some acetaminophen and go back to bed. She'd been down this road before. No sense in getting worked up over a sinus infection. Maybe it wasn't as bizarre as she thought it was when she first woke up this morning.

She was wrong. It didn't go away. Her sense of smell and taste were gone. The sense of déjà vu persisted and became totally disorienting. Beth's klutziness reached new heights. She was constantly tripping over unseen objects or dropping things. She switched to plastic cups instead of glasses, and seriously thought about switching to paper plates. She was nervous that something was wrong both with her, and with the planet in general.

Watching TV made her even more nervous. The news reports were filled with people commenting on secret hand gestures and secret messages from politicians. She was worried because she was left out and didn't know what those gestures and signals were supposed to be. She saw people commenting about lies and fake news, and she didn't understand what they were talking about.

Up until now, she'd been comforted by seeing doctors she knew personally on TV talking about the zombie apocalypse. She realized they had to be imposters. They couldn't possibly be the people she knew and had known and respected for decades. Instead, these imposters who had taken over their bodies were spouting lies. She knew they were lies because the unknown people, the unidentified "they," as in "they say," yet who remain unnamed, talked about the secret signals. "They" told her the experts were liars and repeated that message throughout the airwaves. She knew the experts who she knew personally and trusted wouldn't lie, so either the people on the internet were wrong, or the experts were imposters. It was social media versus people she's known and trusted for decades.

The noise from social media was drowning out the experts. When she finally got back onto social media after being able to reset her passwords, a miracle in itself, Beth saw that a few of her friends on social media were in the "in crowd," and were talking about symbols, hand gestures, secret messages, lies, and fake news. Beth forgot that those so-called friends, who she had not seen or spoken to in decades, had underlying mental health issues. They fed her fear, and she could no longer tell what was true or not. They made her doubt the experts, even though she knew better. But their stories of secret signs, symbols, handshakes, letters, colors, and stories were seductive. Maybe those people could tell her who stole her stuff. As the days went by and her fear escalated, it became impossible to function. She often felt as if she was in a trance. The 24-hour news cycle was relentless. She couldn't get a break for a minute and while George was a great listener, he didn't offer any good advice. Honestly, he was not at all helpful when it came to looking for her missing stuff.

And then came the spiders. There were spiders on the walls all over Beth's house. At first it was one spider. It was giant, the size of a tarantula. It didn't look mean or scary; it hung out on the wall about where one would expect the light switch to be. It was odd looking. It was like one of those cartoonish spiders you see in a Halloween decoration, but this one was real, and it could talk. It didn't say much, just things like, "Hello, Beth" and "It's a little cold in here, can you make it warmer?" It was completely unimpressed by and unafraid of the fox in the sunroom. Fortunately, it was too big for the mouse to eat. It was so big that it could have eaten the mouse. It's a good thing it didn't. Beth hoped the spiders would keep their multiple eyes out for whoever was stealing her stuff. She also thought the spiders could be an early warning sign about the impending robot invasion. Apparently, the zombies were trying to get rid of humanity so the robots could take over.

She had proof that the robots were taking over the planet. For example, there were videos of some Boston Dynamics robots (Atlas, Handle, and Spot) dancing to the song "Do You Love Me" by The Contours. While Beth thoroughly enjoyed watching the robots dance, she realized she should have been scared. How did she know she should have been scared? The people who commented on the social media posts knew something she did not. They were certain the robots were taking over the world and the robots were going to make humans their slaves. With so many humans out of commission due to the alien fog and the zombie apocalypse, the humans should be grateful for the robots which are able to provide humanity with some of the items they needed that the humans weren't able to manufacture or distribute. But the commenters knew better.

Also, it was true some of the robots were completely annoying. There were a pair of robot vehicles that would zoom around Beth's neighborhood at all hours of the day and night, racing down sidewalks, on the wrong side of the road, smashing into pedestrians, scaring the dogs, and being quite loud. They were the right height to do severe damage to a car if they hit it. They were powerful enough to hurt a human being or animal. The police knew the owners, had warned them, and had threatened them. Unfortunately, they lacked the authority to confiscate the robotic cars. The neighbors could do nothing more than complain and ostracize the owners of those robot cars. In the meantime, the Boston Dynamic robots danced, tromped through the snow, and lifted heavy things in the warehouse. She wondered if they knew the robot cars from her neighborhood. Do all robots know each other?

In the meantime, while Beth was contemplating dancing robots, the spiders had babies. Every night, when Beth went to sleep, she could feel baby spiders crawling up and down her right leg. It felt achy. She tried to brush them off, but she wanted to be gentle about it because she didn't want to inadvertently hurt the spiders. Obviously, they were the babies of the big spiders that were all over her wall. She assumed they were in bed with her snuggling as close as they could because they were cold. She couldn't blame them. Still, it felt strange to have baby spiders crawling up and down her leg.

In addition to the spiders, Beth was finding it more challenging to sleep. The bells were ringing constantly. The firetrucks seem to be going up and down her street at least every hour. She even saw Santa Claus driving the truck a few times. But most disconcerting were the strange sounds she couldn't quite tell where they were coming from.

There were the high-pitched sounds like miniature motorcycles going incredibly fast. This happened every single night starting at midnight and didn't stop until three a.m. — zoom, zoom, zoom, getting closer and then fading away. Rarely, but at least occasionally, she would hear a police siren in the distance, and it sounded like it was chasing those motorcycles. Then she would hear the rumble of a car's muffler which was clearly broken or removed. She assumed the drivers thought they sounded cool or it sounded like a muscle car, but it sounded broken.

And the revving of those engines was interrupted regularly by what sounded like gunshots or fireworks. She couldn't see any fireworks, so she assumed it was gunshots. Every night. The gunshots would happen at 2:30 and 3:30 a.m. like clockwork. But, she never heard any sirens. Did no one care there were gunshots every night? She was comforted by the police patrols in her neighborhood. She would see them drive by every thirty minutes. At least, she thought, there's a fighting chance the police would stop any of the nonsense from infringing on her neighborhood. But it wasn't enough to make her comfortable. She couldn't shake the feeling something unbelievably bad was happening.

One morning, right after Christmas, Beth saw on the news that the police had picked up some kids who were drag racing down the highway as part of a gang initiation. They had modified their mufflers to sound like gunshots when they downshifted. They apparently thought it made them look and sound cool. It didn't.

It was cold, dreary, and the ground was covered in dirty gray slushy snow left over from the previous storms. On the one hand, she was impressed the highways had been plowed well enough for those crazy kids to drag race with their gunshot-sounding cars, but on the other hand, everything else just looked dirty. She started dreaming of taking vacations on luxury yachts, sailing around the world, traveling to exotic places, and being waited on hand and foot. Those dreams were unusual for Beth because she usually was hot and would do anything to stay away from a tropical climate.

Beth assumed she must have had the winter blues. Her dreams of luxury yacht tours became her new obsession. She spent more and more of her time daydreaming while sitting in her big pink chair. On motor yacht days, her dream began at a luxury hotel in Boston Harbor. She and her family and friends were having the luxury brunch buffet, and they had taken over the whole restaurant. It was a celebration of some sort, and she assumes it was somewhat work-related since so many of her work colleagues were there as well. And, of course, everyone had brought their dogs who thoroughly enjoyed the gourmet food from the high-end hotel. Docked outside the hotel was a 200-foot motor yacht, and it was hers. It slept twelve, had the most attentive, mature, and competent staff anyone could ever want and Beth loved cruising. Her obsession was quite detailed even if at the same time, it was somewhat discombobulated.

For example, she could describe in detail the suites she and her friends occupied in the luxury hotel, yet on some level even in her daydreams, she recognized it was unusual to sleep in a luxury hotel suite when her luxury yacht was docked fifty feet away. Yet, in her daydream, her suite was gorgeous. The floor-to-ceiling windows overlooked the harbor where she could gaze upon her yacht. There was the most comfortable king-sized bed known to mankind in the room where Beth luxuriated. The marble bathroom had a rainfall shower which was a distinct advantage over the not-quite-as-luxurious albeit not-quite-roughing-it shower on her yacht. And, the suite was spacious. It was close to 2000 square feet. Nothing on a yacht can compare that.

In Beth's daydreams, the first day would begin with the family and friends' brunch. Then, she, her work colleagues/friends, and family chartered a private minibus to tour the city. They started out at Old Ironsides, the oldest active ship in the Navy, walked the Freedom Trail, and ended up at historic Faneuil Hall which was the meeting place prior to the Revolutionary War. While eventually built as a centralized market, it was there where the American patriots met to discuss historic events like the Boston Massacre, the tea party, and other historical events that led to the Revolutionary War. Attached to Faneuil Hall is the Quincy Market marketplace. It's full of shops, restaurants, and is in general, one of Boston's major tourist attractions. Beth always liked to go into the rotunda of the central market and see the sign that used to be posted above a distant cousin's vegetable market hundreds of years ago and now lives in the rotunda. She also dreamed of bringing her friends to eat at the Durgin Park restaurant, now closed, but which had been in continuous operation since the early 1800s.

It was an historically accurate restaurant that featured old New England food. Beth could hear, smell, and taste the food even though the restaurant had been closed for years. She knew her friends, avid history buffs, would thoroughly enjoy going there. She even knew what they would choose to eat. Obviously, it would include clam chowder and cornbread. Someone would get Yankee pot roast. Someone else would get the fried fisherman's platter, someone else would get the prime rib. And Beth would teach them to enjoy grapenut pudding and coffee gelatin. At least, in her dreams she could teach them that.

The next morning would find her wandering with a friend or two throughout the city in search of the best coffee. This part of the dream was always disorienting. On some level, she knew there were five or six great coffee shops within two blocks of the hotel, but she kept wondering, and wandering even farther frantically searching for coffee yet being unable to find out where it was or where she was. That part of the daydream never changed. She was lost in her hometown. But that daydream always resolved itself, and the dream would pick up with Beth and her friends conducting a pizza comparison. Some of Beth's friends would grab slices of pizza in Haymarket Square while others went to the famous Regina's Pizza in the North End. They would meet in the middle to do a taste comparison — a true Bostonian debate.

And then they would sail. They would get on Beth's yacht, pull out into the harbor, and head toward the Cape and the Islands. Along the way, they would see whales and other marine wildlife, and it was gorgeous. Beth could smell the salt air, feel the breeze on her face, hear the waves and the seagulls calling overhead. The ship's crew would constantly offer the freshest fish and seafood to Beth and her guests, who would gorge themselves. Until that point, they had never understood the bounty of seafood available in New England and what Beth meant when she told them that lobster was what you would eat in your bathing suit in the backyard at the pool, and steak was what you would go out to dinner for. Most of them grew up in landlocked places where it was the exact opposite. Beth could see the glee on their faces as they gorged themselves on lobsters, clams, and oysters.

Consistently, the next part of the dream/daydream was where things got strange. The motor yacht would turn into a sailing yacht, and it would be trailing behind all the historical tall ships that paraded through Boston on special occasions. Her yacht would follow them as they circled Cape Cod and the Islands, went through Boston Harbor, and then went through Newport Rhode Island. And there, her sailing yacht would pull into port and turn into a motor yacht. And then, it would sprout wings and fly over the beautiful mansions and estates surrounding Newport. It all seemed normal to her. Then, the flying motor yacht would leave Rhode Island and fly to Salem, Massachusetts, famous for the Salem Witch Trials. They would fly past the House of Seven Gables, over the museums, and they would land in the parking lot of Ye Olde Pepper Company, a store that had been around since the early 1800s and was famous for Gibraltar Rock candies. The candy never spoils, and there is a 100-year-old sample of it in the store. It would be great provisions for the zombie apocalypse.

Throughout the yacht travels, the yacht would expand and shrink in size to fit where it needed to fit. For example, the streets of Salem are incredibly old and narrow. The parking lot in front of the candy store has three spaces, and there is no way a 200-foot yacht could fit down the street or park. Yet, it managed to do so. The distortions of time, space, and geography didn't bother Beth at all. It seemed entirely natural. If she had tried to explain her dreams to anyone, it would've seemed exceedingly weird how on the one hand, she could be so incredibly detailed about what people were eating or what the sidewalks looked like as she walked by, or what the weather was, or what she and her friends were wearing, while at the same time it was entirely logical for her that a ship could transform, fly, drive, and could change sizes.

If Beth were awakened when she was lost and looking for coffee, she would be agitated for the rest of the day. If, however, she let the dream run its course before she woke, or she was woken up at any other point during the dream, she was always happy. She was surrounded by people she loved, she was in places she remembered from her childhood and felt comfortable in, and she was happy to see the confluence of both.

It was so difficult for Beth to be happy these days. She was convinced something was watching her, she was often confused about what she was trying to do, her legs were weak enough that even in her dreams she marveled at her ability to walk any of the places she was dreaming about, and the newest thing was she swore she was covered in spiders. She always had this creepy crawly feeling on her legs, and no matter how much she scratched, she couldn't stop the feeling. She would look and not see anything, but she knew the spiders were there.

Her days of feeling well and having energy to take care of the house were getting fewer and farther between. All she wanted to do was sit in a big pink chair and let her mind wander.

13

JANUARY – THE LANDING

Her travels by yacht were shattered abruptly one day in early January. She had fallen asleep in her big pink chair and was happily dreaming about clam chowder when she heard a crash. One of her mezuzahs, a beautiful glass one, had fallen off the wall and shattered. A mezuzah is a piece of parchment, inscribed with prayers, placed within a decorative case on the door posts of the Jewish home. Two of the main reasons a Jewish person would post a mezuzah are to remind them of their covenant with God, and to let the outside world know this is a Jewish home that has separate rules, beliefs, and traditions. Many Jewish people place a mezuzah on the outside of their front door, while others place them on every doorpost within the house. Beth had collected them for years, more because they were beautiful and she enjoyed them as pieces of traditional art, than for any religious reasons. Each one she had was special to her.

When her favorite glass mezuzah shattered, she could find no reason for it not to still be attached to the wall. She kept hearing the word "Kristallnacht" in her head, repeating over and over as she did her best to sweep up the broken glass. While she wasn't alive yet during Kristallnacht, she was overwhelmed with fear, and could imagine the night of broken glass when the German Nazis came to attack the Jewish businesses. It was visceral. She could feel it as if she had experienced it. And then, a few days later more glass was broken, this time on Capitol Hill when white supremacist zombies rioted. It was the convergence of Beth's nightmares and reality. Beth was terrified.

It appeared the animals were terrified, as well. The squirrels knocked on her sliding glass door and were accompanied by their squirrel families and friends. They asked if they could please seek shelter inside with her. They looked so afraid, she couldn't say no. The fox came back with some stray kits and asked if they could stay as well. Of course, Beth said yes. She was grateful for her persistence on the apocalypse planning because she knew she had enough food and supplies for all of the animals who were afraid to remain outside.

Armageddon was in full force. There were riots; fire and flood at the same time in the same place; deaths from some strange virus happening faster than people could bury the dead; storms that hurtled snow, sleet, rain, and freezing fog at the same time; fox, deer, bears, coyotes, and buzzards wandering through major cities; snowstorms in places that had never seen snow; power outages; water shortages and more. It was as if all the rules of "polite" society had disappeared. People stopped following safety measures. Cars drove on the wrong side of the street. Trucks with snowplow blades drove around in circles while the metal of the blades threw sparks on the sidewalks in the streets and started fires. Yet, they never picked up their blades. Gangs of men walked in a row putting their hands in buckets and throwing things on the ground. Much of the country was covered in ice, the invisible kind people didn't see until it was too late, and they fell on it. The ice was merciless. In addition to making streets and sidewalks and driveways lethal skating rinks, it hung like daggers from rooftops, cracked water pipes, and the broken pipes caused more ice. The ice was taking over.

At the same time, the zombies gave up all pretense of trying to live peacefully with their neighbors. Armed with ridiculous clothing and Halloween costumes, they rioted, engaged people in hand-to-hand combat, and attacked with bear spray. They engaged in murder and mayhem and attacked people at home, at work, and in random places throughout the community. The zombies did their best to take over. But the zombies overplayed their hand. Even their friends vilified them on TV and social media. No one thought they were fun, benign, or right anymore. And people looked for ways to rid the planet of zombies.

That was about the time the aliens and the human scientists teamed up. The aliens had proven to themselves they were able to live among the humans relatively peacefully but the humans needed help protecting themselves from themselves and from the zombies. So, they taught the human scientists how to make an antidote from the alien fog to combat the zombie disease. The aliens taught the scientists how to stick probes up the humans' noses to determine if the humans were infected with the zombie disease. Then, the aliens taught the human scientists how to administer the antidote by sticking needles in the humans' arms. It looked like every horror movie featuring the aliens as bad guys that had ever been shown on earth. This time, however, the aliens were the good guys. But the zombies fought back. They partnered with human conspiracy theorists and tried to hijack social media. They did their best to tell humans that the scientists were lying and the antidote would kill them. Some people believed them.

Then the zombies flaunted their "proof" that they were right and the aliens and scientists were wrong. They gathered in large groups again. Their riots spread disease throughout the country. Their families turned against them. Zombies kept fighting, but the aliens and the scientists were slowly gaining an advantage. And for the first time in more than a year, there was hope the world could get back to "normal." The scientists smiled. They had known this would happen all along. The identification of zombies threw Beth into a tizzy. She had no idea who was real and who was an imposter.

Beth felt as if she was stuck in the spin cycle of a dryer. Objects of different colors, shapes, sizes, and textures were spinning around her like a tornado. She was stuck in the barrel of the dryer, spinning, hot, trapped, overwhelmed, and completely unable to escape. She was terrified. The outside world was spinning. The humans, zombies, and aliens were engaged in a war of words Beth couldn't understand. She told the mouse she felt like her brain was being fried. She started to feel colors. At night, when the police cars drove by with their blue lights flashing, Beth felt cold. When the fire trucks and ambulances passed her house with their red lights flashing, she felt hot. The same was true when she saw colors on TV. The world was spinning out of control, and Beth honestly felt like she was losing her mind.

Amidst all this spinning and colors and heat and cold, Beth was entirely discombobulated and disoriented. Every time she looked out her windows, she saw fog. That freezing mist she had seen for almost a year surrounded her house. She was too disoriented to recognize that it was protecting her. Instead, as she stayed in her house, surrounded by fog, she was overwhelmed by the hands and faces of the zombies who were trying to break through the fog to get into her house. They were trapped in the mist and desperate to break into her house. They started flashing red and blue strobe lights to confuse her. And the colors and the noise and the lights and the sound and the temperature and the yelling surrounding the zombies was more than Beth could handle. The thing that kept her from losing her mind completely was the comfort of being surrounded by friends and relatives who had passed away. They countered the red and blue lights with white lights of their own and told her she was safe, she was loved, and she was protected. For brief moments when they surrounded her, Beth felt as though there was a possibility the spin cycle might stop. She would do anything, anything to make it end. Her brain and her soul couldn't handle the tumult anymore.

One of the more mundane things was one of the most annoying for Beth. She became completely obsessed with using the bathroom. She would walk into the bathroom, pull down her pants, sit on the toilet, forget what she was going to do, pull up her pants, wash her hands, and walk out of the bathroom. She did this every thirty minutes all day long. Occasionally she would remember what she was supposed to do when she sat on the toilet. The mouse, the fox, George, and "everyone" else who lived in her house were worried. Her behavior puzzled even the zombies who still looked through her windows. Beth was annoyed.

Her bladder was always uncomfortable. But she couldn't remember that she needed to use the toilet, nor could she remember she had just been in the bathroom without using it.

It was around this time she realized she was seeing things that only a few other people could see. She saw strangely dressed people marching around Capitol Hill again. Clearly, they saw the same bears invading the Capitol that she did. If they didn't, why were they using bear spray to fight off the navy blue bears she saw on TV? Beth had no idea these were zombie-induced hallucinations.

All Beth knew was she had to flee. She knew she had to leave her house. She wasn't sure where she was going, but she knew she had to escape. It wasn't a case of running away *to* something, it was a case of running away *from*... She had lost her fear of the unknown and replaced it with the unidentified fears within her own house. She's tried to flee multiple times over the past few months. She never gets far. Usually, she gets lost in the cul-de-sac outside her house and runs in circles. If she ever gets farther down the street, she usually trips and falls down at the next intersection. Fortunately, her neighbors watch out for her and help her to get home every time. They always are kind and gentle, but she's terrified of them. The ones who make her feel safe are the faceless, nondescript, navy blue sweater–wearing ones. Sometimes, the flashing blue lights would come to her house and she would be freezing cold. Other times, the flashing red lights would come to her house and she would feel their heat. Throughout all of this was the unrelenting fear. Yet, somewhere, in the back of her mind, there was a piece of her trying to save itself. She couldn't find the words to describe it, but instinctively, she knew part of herself was trying to save her.

One day, the part of her that still remained drove Beth to take a walk to the local park. Unfortunately, it was the middle of the night in the middle of winter. There was a hypothermia alert issued by the local government, but Beth didn't know, nor could she have understood. She was determined to go to the local park and to go to that local park *now*. When she got there, she was surprised to see there was a carousel with brightly painted animals, bright lights, upbeat carousel-type music, and everything one would expect from the good old-fashioned carousel Beth had grown up with. Next to it was a small snack stand that sold ice cream, hot dogs, and popcorn. Beth could smell the popcorn and the hotdogs. The park was filled with children dressed in brightly colored summer clothes and dogs of all sizes wearing T-shirts with clowns on them. The squirrels, the mouse and his friends, and the fox were romping around among the kids and the dogs, hoping for popcorn or hotdogs to fall. The dogs were licking the ice cream cones right out of the children's hands.

Much to her surprise, Beth saw that one of the dogs was pulling a red flyer wagon, like the ones Beth had had as a child. It was filled with hundreds of people who lived in the plants in Beth's sunroom. They were laughing, singing, and dancing to the band playing in the corner of the wagon. Everyone was happy, playful, and clearly enjoying themselves. Beth watched as the carousel expanded into a full carnival with rides, games, and most importantly, cotton candy. The kids walked around with enormous stuffed animals as prizes. Even the people who lived among the plants had teeny tiny stuffed animal prizes loaded into their wagon. The dogs had bones. The squirrels had paper cones filled with nuts, as did the mice. And the fox ran by with an entire string of hotdogs and a big grin on his face. Beth felt a sense of overwhelming joy to be part of this celebration. She had no idea what they were celebrating, but still, she was thrilled to be part of it. She ran laughing and smiling and dancing through the park, dressed in shorts and a T-shirt and barefoot, and was completely happy. She didn't notice when the snow began to fall. She didn't notice that no one else was in the park. She didn't notice it was the middle of the night. She didn't notice there was no carnival. The only things in the dark, empty, bitterly cold park were Beth, the picnic table, and a few snow-covered benches.

The next thing Beth knew, she felt a flash of overwhelming heat. She felt rather than saw, red. Looking closely, she saw a big red truck with red lights; it rumbled as if it were hungry, and she could feel the heat coming off of it in waves. Next to the red pulled up blue. The blue was smaller and colder than the red. Before Beth had a chance to puzzle out the difference between the sizes of the red and the blue and the hot and the cold, bears jumped out of both the red and the blue. Two of the bears carried big fuzzy blankets and slowly walked toward her. She couldn't understand what they were saying, but they clearly were trying to communicate with her. They spoke softly and gently and the two with the blankets approached her from the front. They did their best to keep her focus on them. It worked, and Beth was completely unaware the other bears were making a circle around her. She was not afraid of the bears in front of her, and she was feeling a bit cold, so the blankets intrigued her.

She looked down at her own bare feet and was surprised she wasn't wearing shoes. The blanket-carrying bears were wearing boots. The shorter of the two bears reached out his arm and offered his blanket to her. Beth took it, wrapped it around her shoulders, and realized she was quite cold. The taller bear reached out his hand to her, but Beth was too afraid to take it. She started shivering. Then got scared, really scared. She didn't know where she was, and she didn't understand why she was surrounded by red and blue and bears. She felt trapped, and knew she needed to escape. She didn't know where she was going, but she knew she needed to be away from there. She needed to be away from the threatening bears.

The shorter bear must have sensed her fear. He motioned with his hands for all of the other bears to back away. He took the blanket from the second bear, placed it on the ground, sat down next to it, and patted it to encourage Beth to sit down on it next to him. He was comforting for Beth. He kept speaking in low tones, he was sitting down, and while his company of bears was watching and waiting and aware, he felt safe. Beth sat down next to him on the nice warm blanket. She didn't realize he was sitting in the cold snow. He kept making soothing sounds which Beth did not understand, but which communicated to her in a way she knew she was going to be safe. He reached his hand out to her, and she took it.

With some difficulty, he got off the ground, and helped Beth get off the ground as well. He held her hand as they walked to the little red truck she hadn't noticed. He knocked on the doors, and the bears inside reached out their hands to Beth. She was scared, so the blue bear who was with her got into the truck first, without ever letting go of her hand. She followed him in. He pointed to the bed that was in the truck, and he helped her into it. The two other bears in the truck smiled at her. She was so tired; the fear and the cold had exhausted her. As confused as she was, she knew she was safe. And the bear who had brought her the blanket was there, and he kept holding her hand and making those comforting sounds. One of the other bears got into the front of the truck, and the second bear stayed behind with Beth and the blanket-bearing bear. He shut the door, the truck started up, and it drove down the street.

Beth had no idea where she was, she had no idea where she was going, she had no idea why she was in a truck full of bears, but she was so exhausted she fell asleep.

She woke up to a terrifying sight. The red truck had parked in a cave, bears wearing white coats flung open the back door of the truck, and they pulled Beth's bed with her in it right out of the truck. They were yammering at each other and at Beth in some foreign language she couldn't possibly understand, and she became terrified again. She thrashed around under her blanket and realized she couldn't move off of the bed. For some reason, she couldn't move her arms and legs well. She let out a bloodcurdling scream out of sheer terror. It was clear she was totally panicking. Fortunately, her bear "friend" took her hand and made those calming noises again. Some of the sounds sounded like what the other bears were saying, and Beth still couldn't understand them, but she felt safe with that particular bear. He held her hand as the white-coated bears pushed her bed farther into the cave.

At the back of the cave was a door. The team of bears pushed her bed through the door, and it was like she entered an alternate universe. It was hellacious. Beth was lying on her back on a moving bed, and the painfully bright lights in the ceiling were shining directly down on her like laser beams. People were yelling everywhere, bears were pushing her bed, robots and blinking and beeping machines were trying to eat the people. The machines were reaching their arms and tentacles into people's throats and on their wrists and over their heads and the machines had TVs on them and the TV monitors kept beeping and clicking and showing strange pictures of lines going up and down and numbers flashing. The people who were not being eaten by machines were entirely faceless and unidentifiable. Many of them were making strange crying noises. Creatures in yellow or white spacesuits with missing faces were marching up and down the hallways and leaning over the people who were being eaten by machines. Beth again tried in vain to move her arms and legs, but they felt so weak she couldn't move them at all. Throughout all of the chaos and the terror, the calming bear never let go of Beth's hand. He kept her grounded.

The calming bear told her that he needed to leave but his friends would take care of her. He told her she was safe. She trusted him, and she believed him, so she was able to remain calm even though she still was scared. Then, many bears, all wearing white coats, surrounded her. They were asking questions she didn't understand, they were shining lights in her eyes, they put a vinyl cuff on her arm, and it kept squeezing her until it hurt. Then it would stop squeezing for a few seconds and give her some relief, but after a few seconds it squeezed her again. They put what looked like a soda cap with a string on it on her finger. It had a red light inside. It kept flashing numbers in blue on the top. Everybody seemed extremely interested in those blue numbers. She didn't like it, so she took it off and threw it across the room. Immediately after she did that, she felt something cold on her wrist. She didn't have time to examine it, however, because even more bears came in and started doing things to her.

Beth grew more agitated by all of the people poking and prodding at her and subjecting her to a barrage of questions. She knew she had to escape. She knew she had to flee; she didn't know where she was going, she knew she had to get out of where she was. She tried to sit up but couldn't. It was then she noticed her left arm had a bracelet on it and the bracelet was attached to the bed. She couldn't flee, she couldn't run away, she was completely trapped. She did the only thing she could. She screamed.

She was disoriented and terrified, and yet the bears kept doing things to her. They poked her with sharp things. She thought she saw blood. They put rubber tubes up her nose that went around her chin and attached to a strange-looking machine. She felt cold air going up her nose, and strangely, while it completely terrified her, on some level, it somewhat calmed her down. Not calm enough, apparently, though. One of the bears took a needle attached to a plastic test tube, stuck it in Beth's arm, and taped it there. The worst part was, apparently the bear couldn't find the right place on Beth's arm to stick the sharp needle, so she tied a horribly tight rubber hose around Beth's upper arm, poking Beth with the needle, then hit Beth's forearm to try to find a better place to stick the needle. Even Beth could tell the bear was getting frustrated. Beth was angry. She was really angry. Why was the bear getting frustrated when Beth was the one being repeatedly stabbed with a sharp object?

After an eternity, the bear finally got the needle into and taped where she wanted it. Then, she took a tall metal pole with a plastic bag of water hanging from it and hooked that hose to the plastic tube in Beth's arm. It was cold. Beth could feel it running through her whole body and it felt miserable. And then, another bear came with a small glass vial and yet another needle. Beth screamed again. And then, as the bear used the needle to take the liquid out of the vial and squeezed it into the tube coming out of Beth's arm, Beth fell silent.

Immediately before she fell silent, inside her head, she heard her brain scream: "Help! I can't move! I can't move my arms or legs!" But since the scream was inside her head, no one knew, and no one responded. Beth was paralyzed, literally. Her muscles stiffened and became rigid. She felt she was locked inside her completely unresponsive body and trapped in this terrifying version of hell, surrounded by faceless bears, needles, and machines trying to eat her alive. Even worse than that, she was speaking in gibberish and had lost all language ability. No one could understand anything she was saying, no one understood her fear, and no one understood she was totally paralyzed.

Fortunately, although Beth couldn't see him, someone *was* listening. A new bear came running into the room. While he, too, was faceless and wearing a white lab coat, she could see his fur was gray and thinning. He clearly was older than the other bears. He looked in Beth's eyes, gripped her hand, glanced at the machines, and then, in a booming, authoritative voice looked at the other bears in the room and asked, "Who the f*ck thought it was a good idea to give her haloperidol?" Beth had no way of knowing this new gray-haired bear was the only one who understood exactly what was going on. All she knew was that after he threw all of the other bears out, he lightly touched Beth's shoulder, looked in her eyes, and promised she would be safe with him. "I'm in charge of your case now," he reassured her. "And I understand what you're going through and I will help you to the best of my ability." He didn't have the heart to tell her that he couldn't totally fix it. But at least Beth's terror lessened.

He went out into the hallway, found two bears who had not been with Beth earlier, and led the way as they wheeled Beth into a peaceful, serene, safe room. They gently lifted her into the most comfortable bed she'd ever been in. When she looked up, the overhead lights were behind the screen of pretty flowers in bright, cheerful, primary colors. It not only gave her something to look at, but it screened the harsh overhead lights, so they didn't hurt her eyes. Her room was on the third floor with huge picture windows looking out over the snow-covered landscape.

What seemed like an eternity later, Beth fell into a dreamless sleep. She had no idea how long it lasted, but when she awoke, she saw her mother, her father, her sister, and her sister's two dogs peering in through the doorway of her room. She didn't recognize them, and couldn't identify them, but she knew she was safe. Everybody was acting oddly around her, and she was puzzled. As she struggled to figure out what was going on, the two dogs launched themselves at her, jumped into her bed, and rolled all over her and licked her face while madly wagging their tails. Their joy was evident. She immediately felt happy and comfortable, even though she was still disoriented.

Looking out the door, she saw the white-coated bears, including her favorite gray-furred one, talking to the people she recognized as her family. She cried because she hadn't seen them in forever, and she had been so scared. Briefly, in a rare moment of clarity, she wondered how on earth her family knew where she was and how to find her, and she was completely flabbergasted that the dogs had gotten to her as well. She couldn't remember why that was strange, but she knew that it was. She was glad to be less foggy-headed and less terrified, even if for a short while.

What Beth did not know was the nice bear that calmed her down in the park had gone back to her neighborhood after he brought her to safety. Beth wasn't aware he had escorted her all the way to hospital. She had been completely out of it. He, however, didn't like that the hospital referred to her as "Jane Doe," so he made it his mission to find out who she was. He slowly drove up and down the streets near the park where he had found her. Beth's neighbors, suspecting something unusual was going on since it was rare for police to be driving up and down the street came out of their houses, even though it was the middle of the night, with winter coats over their pajamas and slippers. He described what Beth looked like, and some of the neighbors knew where she lived. They took him to her house. Fortunately, other neighbors knew how to get in touch with her family. It was an entire community getting together to keep Beth safe. She knew none of this. But Beth was lucky, or, as lucky as one could be in such a horrible situation. Her family was found, and they were able to get to her and help her before she was sent somewhere where it would be virtually impossible for her family to ever find her.

Instead, the gray-furred bear was able to care for Beth and reverse the side effects of the medicine she had been given. She was able to go home, although due to the zombie apocalypse things were vastly different than anyone would have wanted.

Her family brought her home, and Beth was thrilled to be back. She was happy to see George, the mouse, the fox, the boy and girl, and the diminutive people. They were happy to see her, as well. Much to her surprise, the dogs paid no attention to any of Beth's roommates. But, Beth's surprise was tempered by her gratefulness that no one was going to fight.

Apparently, the white-coated bears had convinced Beth's family that Beth needed to self-isolate alone at home to protect everyone from zombies. It seemed ridiculous to them and to Beth since they had all been together the day before, but Beth was far too exhausted to argue, and her family was far too scared. It was possible the zombies had converted her while she was living with the white-coated bears. They had allowed her family to take her home and to enter her house for fifteen minutes while wearing yellow spacesuits with clear plastic masks covering their eyes, gloves covering their hands, and blue booties covering their shoes. The refrigerator was stocked with food that didn't need to be cooked at all or could be microwaved, protein shakes, and plenty of good desserts. The house was spotlessly cleaned. It was obvious Beth's mother had scrubbed it top to bottom. There were new video screens in every room. Beth's sister explained that it was so she could talk to them whenever she wanted and all she had to do was say, "Call Mom, Dad, or my sister," and they would show up on the screens. And then the timer marking the 15-minute limit went off. Beth's family and the dogs waved goodbye and left.

Beth felt much calmer and less afraid than she had for months. She was pleased to see her family had remembered to restock her Diet Coke®. Grabbing one, she slowly made her way to her bedroom to take a rest. While mentally she felt better, her muscles, particularly her right leg, felt incredibly weak, and she felt dizzy and off balance. She got into bed, turned on the TV, and promptly fell asleep.

The next morning, she woke up ravenous. She got out of bed, stood up, and made her way to the bathroom. It sounds like a simple enough task, but she was thrilled to not be dizzy and to be able to maintain her balance. Then, while sidestepping to put her toothbrush back in its holder, she tripped over the bathmat. Fortunately, she was able to catch herself before she fell. Moving more gingerly than before, she walked into the kitchen and was thrilled to see a freezer bag with already sliced bagels right there on the counter. She opened the cabinet to take out a dish and noticed there already were dishes neatly stacked on the kitchen counter below the cabinet they usually were stored in. It was much easier for her to reach the dishes this way, she thought. She didn't have to stretch to try to reach them. "I wonder who thought of this," she mused. She carefully placed a bagel on one of the dishes and rummaged through the refrigerator to see what she might want to top the bagel with. She found veggie cream cheese and lox, her favorite combination. Even better, someone had opened the usually-impossible-to-open vacuum-sealed package of lox and put it in a much easier-to-open freezer bag. She was thrilled. Today, it was easy for her to make her own breakfast and she was hungry enough to eat it.

Recently, in the past two months or so, her appetite had changed. Some days, she wanted nothing except Diet Coke®. She could barely choke down a protein shake, and even then, it was the easy-to-open cardboard ones. The bottles, with their safety seals, proved to be too much of a challenge to be worth it. Then, on other days, she ate everything in sight. She grew particularly fond of cookies and ice cream sandwiches, not usually her food of choice. It was unusual, but since she had it, she ate it. Occasionally, she would supplement with snacks she found in her pre-zombie apocalypse preparation stash. In general, however, her nutrition was abysmal.

It was interesting that even though some days consisted entirely of the snack food, cookie, and ice cream diet, Beth still lost a lot of weight. She had always struggled with her weight and had been on perpetual diets, so she certainly was not displeased when her clothes were too big. She saw nothing wrong with a significant weight loss over a short period of time, even though she wasn't trying. It was the polar opposite of the way she'd been her whole life. Normally, she joked that she could gain weight by watching someone else eat a piece of cake, and seemingly without effort, the pounds were dropping off of her. For the first time in her life, she was too skinny. It never dawned on her that this could be a problem.

She also wasn't worried about how stiff her muscles were becoming. It would take her more than a few minutes after she'd wake up to make her muscles "warm up." At least, she thinks that's the term. She never was much of an athlete, but she remembered hearing stories of how one should stretch to loosen one's muscles before exercising. She never did it, but at least she remembered it. She started keeping her four-pronged cane next to the bed in case she needed to go to the bathroom in the middle of the night. She wasn't sure how to prevent a fall while her muscles were so stiff and weak. In the past few months, she physically got a lot worse. She chalked it up to lack of exercise since the weather had been too bad to walk outside much.

Today was a good day, however. She was energized by her breakfast, thrilled to accompany it with a nice cold Diet Coke®, and for the first time in a long time, she was not terrified and agitated. She still was exhausted, however, so she brought her bagel and Diet Coke® back to bed and decided to eat there. All in all, she was content, although she was a bit puzzled. In the back of her mind, she remembered something about bears wearing white doctor/lab coats, and she had this odd feeling she had seen her parents, her sister, and the dogs. But, she couldn't tell whether it was memory or fantasy. Everything seemed fuzzy. After eating her bagel and finishing her Diet Coke®, she fell asleep, so she didn't ponder it for long.

Her family, on the other hand, was horrified. They had been horrified by the condition of the house, terrified at Beth's physical appearance, and completely appalled by how mentally "out of it" she was. She was detached from and unaware of how bad things had gotten. They knew that for the next two weeks, however, they were unable to stay with her due to the chance she had become a victim of the zombie apocalypse. No one else could come in, either. While she had been tested, the fear was the testing had been done too early, and the zombie antibodies hadn't shown up yet. No one was allowed in the house. So they did their best. They visited through the sliding glass door, and they left food in her garage. They talked to her through the fancy screens in her house. It was devastating for them. They felt entirely helpless. Their consolation was Beth was entirely oblivious to any problems.

Sometime during the second week, when they were able to see her in person by outdoor visiting, they realized Beth didn't recognize who they were. She never addressed them by name, never directed any conversation to them, and seemed scared of them. She did, however, always recognize the dogs and was thrilled to see them. Even that was worrisome to Beth's family. The dogs were treating her differently. They were exceedingly protective of her and guarded her, even against her own family. One of them was always either sitting on her or sitting in front of her as if on patrol. They would switch shifts to never leave her alone. Once Beth went back into her house after the visits, the dogs would stand by the door guarding the house from the outside. They had to be picked up and carried to the car to get them to leave. The dogs clearly knew something was wrong, even more than the human family did, and certainly more than Beth herself did. Beth was beginning to understand something was wrong.

14

FEBRUARY – THE CRASH

Something's wrong. Something's really, really, wrong. The poltergeists and spiders are merciless. The exhaustion is constant. Beth has no energy. Fear is strangling her. She's totally forgotten that it is darkest before the dawn. She feels trapped within her own mind and as though part of her soul is struggling to get out of her brain, but it can't. The struggle is exhausting, the fear is overwhelming, and the confusion has taken over entirely. Beth can't find a way out.

Beth no longer is comforted by the people, aliens, and animals that have been watching her. She is terrified all the time. She's alone and lonely. Her body no longer responds the way she wants it to. She's tired of tripping over things, she's tired of tripping over nothing except her own feet. She's tired of not being able to use her right arm, and she's tired of dropping things from her right hand. She's tired of the constant noise: voices, cars, gunshots, fireworks, bells, and the music running through her brain. It never stops. The noise is merciless.

Strangers watch her through the mirrors. Watching, always watching, and commenting on whatever it is she's doing wrong. Is what she sees real? Is it fake? Has she been lied to? Is she getting magic signals through the TV? Was there really a storm coming? What kind of storm? Real or allegorical? Was there something mystical about the number seventeen? Her head was spinning. With her own eyes, she saw people watching her through the mirrors, zombies looking through the window, she had flown on spaceships, she saw animals everywhere, even in her house. Recently, she was obsessed with the movies. Sometimes she felt the movies were playing only for her, but she watched them intently. She searched for secret messages in them. She searched for a clue about what she was supposed to do next.

And the noise got worse. The sounds got more relentless. The noise and the sounds blocked out her thoughts. She couldn't concentrate, she couldn't make sense, and she couldn't make it stop. She wanted it to stop.

Beth felt like her brain was disintegrating. She knows she's no longer who she used to be. She feels unhinged and ungrounded. She feels as though she's fallen down a rabbit hole. She believes that reality as we know it isn't real. Instead, she feels as though we are operating in parallel universes. Or perhaps we're stuck inside the Matrix. Maybe this is a simulated reality. Maybe she holds the key? It's impossible to tell who's a zombie, who's an alien, who is real, and who's an imposter. Beth feels her head is going to explode.

And then the noise gets louder. It's more intense. It's completely overtaking her mind. It's morphing into a type of buzzing that nothing else can get through. The animals, zombies, aliens, people, spider, the movies in the mirrors, and the flashing on the TV are pummeling her. Her brain can't keep up anymore.

She gets in her car and starts to drive. She wants to get away from it all. She's not sure where she's headed. Vaguely, she seems to be headed toward the mountains. Deep in the vestiges of her soul, she remembers the stories of the "school on high." In Hebrew, that phrase has come to mean "heaven." She's not afraid to die. In Judaism, there is no hell, and heaven has an open-door policy. Anyone righteous belongs in heaven.

As she drives, in the vestiges of her mind she remembers discussions about life and death with beliefs and stories passed generation to generation. She's not afraid to die. She's not afraid of the world to come.

She's not even thinking of that. Were she to think of that, she would be comforted because of her beliefs and the words she had read.

In *Moment Magazine*, Professor A. J. Levine highlighted a variety of Jewish afterlife concepts, ranging from the traditional expectation of bodily resurrection to the belief in living on through descendants, and even a version of heaven that might favor lox and bagels over traditional celestial symbols. Additionally, a particular perspective within Judaism, as explained by Rabbi Shmuley Boteach in his book *The Wolf Shall Lie with the Lamb: The Messiah in Hassidic Thought*, views heaven as a temporary station for souls awaiting reunification with their bodies during the messianic age, a concept distinct from the cycle of rebirth found in Hinduism, as this reunification is envisioned as a singular event.

But on a conscious level, Beth was not thinking of any of this. She wanted a way out. Any way out. So, she kept driving. Beth lost all sense of time, space, or place. She kept driving.

The road stretched out before her and the voices got louder, and the noise more intense, and no matter how far she drove, she couldn't make it stop. The suffering was unbearable.

Beth glanced over at the passenger seat and was surprised to see her neighbor. As usual, he was totally nondescript and wearing his favorite bulky navy-blue sweater. He said nothing to her but reached out and put his hand on her shoulder. Together, they rode in silence. After an eternity, he pointed to the next exit up ahead. The sign said nothing more than "exit here." Beth took the exit and drove directly into bright white lights, an overwhelming feeling of being loved, and an overall sense of peace. And it was good.

EPILOGUE

The main character, Beth, suffers from Lewy body dementia. Lewy body dementia is a serious illness that sometimes can be mistaken for Alzheimer's disease, Parkinson's disease, or something else.

Lewy body dementia (LBD) is the second most common type of progressive dementia after Alzheimer's disease. LBD is not a rare disease. It affects more than a million people and their families in the United States alone. Because LBD symptoms may closely resemble other more commonly known disorders like Alzheimer's disease, it is currently widely under-diagnosed.[1]

What is a Lewy body? Protein deposits, called Lewy bodies, develop in nerve cells in the brain regions involved in thinking, memory, and movement (motor control). Lewy body dementia causes a progressive decline in mental abilities. People with Lewy body dementia may experience visual hallucinations and changes in alertness and attention. Other effects include Parkinson's disease-like signs and symptoms such as rigid muscles, slow movement, and tremors.[2] In this book, the Lewy body protein deposits are represented by the sea glass. Beth's symptoms increase as the amount of sea glass increases. Lewy body proteins somewhat resemble the shape of a thumbprint cookie or sea glass although clearly on a microscopic level. While this book is fictional but based in science, in this case, the author has taken some artistic license.

In real life, the presence of Lewy bodies does not necessarily mean a person has Lewy body dementia. Many scientists consider Lewy body dementia and Parkinson's disease to fall on a spectrum because there is a demonstrable presence of Lewy bodies in both diseases. However, there are clinical and practical differences in the way the diseases manifest and progress.[3] Fluctuating cognition and visual hallucinations are a hallmark of Lewy body dementia. Signs and symptoms can be consistent with Parkinson's disease, such as tremors, a shuffling gait, and falls. One distinguishing feature is the profound sensitivity to certain medications, including antipsychotics like Haldol.[4]

Visual hallucinations occur in two-thirds of patients with Lewy body dementia, but they are rare in patients with Alzheimer's disease. In fact, visual hallucinations in dementia have an 83 percent positive predictive value for Lewy body. REM sleep behavior disorder is another strange but intriguing manifestation. A person with a healthy brain will not move much during REM sleep, but a person with Lewy body dementia might kick, punch, or thrash about the bed, much to the consternation of his or her partner.[5]

As previously noted, Lewy body dementia can look a lot like Parkinson's disease. Imaging studies are not usually helpful in making the diagnosis, even with identification of Lewy bodies. Lewy bodies are found in Parkinson's disease, Lewy body dementia, supranuclear palsy, Parkinson's disease with dementia, and multiple system atrophy. Their presence on autopsy is always considered pathologically significant.[6]

Throughout the book, there are examples of symptoms commonly found in people with Lewy body dementia. One such example is George, the character who always stands by the door. In reality, George is a coat rack with a hat on top, overcoat hanging on it, and an umbrella in the attached umbrella stand. Beth experiences a visual misperception and identifies the coat rack as a person. Another example is the character of the fox. The fox is a metal plant stand in which one would place a potted plant. It is shaped like a colorful fox, but there is a large hole in the back where the pot would be inserted, and it most certainly is not alive. The bear in Beth's bedroom is a pile of clean laundry. It is rotund, it does resemble a bear, but it is not alive, and it is not a bear. The bears that helped Beth when she wandered to the park were police officers, EMTs, and medical staff from the hospital. Because their bodies are shapeless under uniforms, lab coats, etc. and they were wearing protective masks and gloves, it was easy for someone with Lewy body dementia to mistake them for bears. The little boy and girl are 36-inch-tall decorative sculptures that hold a bottle of wine and a dish. They are not alive.

The poltergeist explained some of the physical Parkinson's-like symptoms common to people with Lewy body dementia. Beth's difficulty in placing dinnerware on a placemat was blamed on the poltergeist moving the mat as opposed to Beth's declining spatial recognition and movement abilities. Additionally, the poltergeist was "responsible" for moving Beth's things when in reality, she didn't remember where she put them. The Parkinson's-like symptoms repeat throughout the book with Beth's stumbling or dropping things.

Beth suffers from Capgras syndrome, a delusion which is a temporary belief that a family member, caregiver, or location has been replaced by an identical imposter.[7] The author has taken some artistic liberty by substituting the location with objects being imposters in Beth's delusions. Delusions are false beliefs. They often are mistaken for hallucinations.

Beth also suffers from hallucinations. Hallucinations may be one of the first symptoms, and they often recur. They may include seeing shapes, animals or people that aren't there. Sound (auditory), smell (olfactory), or touch (tactile) hallucinations are possible.[8] There are many examples of hallucinations throughout the book. One such example is the passenger who joined Beth in the taxi on the way to the hotel in Las Vegas. There was no other person in the taxi.

Additionally, Beth suffers from REM sleep disturbance. That also is typical of somebody with Lewy body dementia. She experiences exceedingly vivid dreams, and often acts them out in her sleep.

A final symptom is prosopagnosia, the inability to recognize faces. Beth also had trouble recognizing faces, which is why many of the characters were described as faceless creatures. The faceless creatures also served the second purpose. This book was written during a pandemic, and people wore masks. Masks, especially when combined with sunglasses, totally obscured people's faces. So, during the pandemic, while the inability to recognize faces is indeed a symptom of Lewy body dementia, it was a moot point. No one could identify anyone's faces.

The zombie apocalypse represents a few different things. First, it represents COVID-19, but more importantly, it represents people's behaviors during a pandemic. Some of the zombie behavior was more unusual than the behavior of someone with dementia. There are examples of this interwoven throughout the book. One such example is the belief in secret signs and symbols and conspiracy. Those beliefs are similar to the delusional thinking one would expect in a person with Lewy body dementia, and they were common among certain people during the pandemic. Consequently, this behavior was attributed to zombies in the book.

The squirrels are real. They happily eat every annual plant they can get their little paws on. Fortunately, they do not come into the house. The mouse also is real. It's primary contribution to this book was to scurry around the house evading traps until it decided to vacate the premises.

[1] https://www.lbda.org/what-is-lbd/ accessed 4/2/2021

[2] https://www.mayoclinic.org/diseases-conditions/lewy-body-dementia/symptoms-causes/syc-20352025 accessed 4/2/2021

[3] Simmons, Steven P., William E. Mansbach, and Jodi L. Lyons. *Brain Health as You Age: a Practical Guide to Maintenance and Prevention*. Lanham, MD: Rowman & Littlefield, 2018. Page 56

[4] Simmons, Steven P., William E. Mansbach, and Jodi L. Lyons. *Brain Health as You Age: a Practical Guide to Maintenance and Prevention*. Lanham, MD: Rowman & Littlefield, 2018. Page 58

[5] Simmons, Steven P., William E. Mansbach, and Jodi L. Lyons. *Brain Health as You Age: a Practical Guide to Maintenance and Prevention*. Lanham, MD: Rowman & Littlefield, 2018. page 58

[6] Simmons, Steven P., William E. Mansbach, and Jodi L. Lyons. *Brain Health as You Age: a Practical Guide to Maintenance and Prevention*. Lanham, MD: Rowman & Littlefield, 2018. page 59

[7] https://www.lbda.org/capgras-syndrome-in-dlb-associated-with-anxiety-and-hallucinations/ accessed 4/8/2021.

[8] https://www.mayoclinic.org/diseases-conditions/lewy-body-dementia/symptoms-causes/syc-20352025 accessed 4/8/2021

Acknowledgements

No book is written in a vacuum or without extensive support for the author. I am fortunate to have a talented, kind, supportive village that provides me with the opportunity to write!

Thank you to Rand-Smith and their team for all of their hard work in making this book become a reality.

I am grateful to my literary agent, Diane Nine, as always, for her expertise, unwavering support, and friendship.

Thank you to my parents, Linda and Ed Lyons, and sister, Shari for their encouragement, entertainment, and use of their houses when I needed a change of scenery.

Thanks to my friends for their encouragement, care, and literal feeding. I appreciate your constant supply of emotional support, checking in, and home-baked goodies!

Thank you to the dedicated clinicians and researchers who work tirelessly to care for people with dementia and strive to find a cure. I always learn from you.

Finally, to those who are living with dementia, thank you for being the inspiration for this book.

--Jodi Lyons

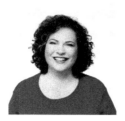

Jodi L. Lyons, Chief Care Officer at CareBrains (www.carebrains.com), is an eldercare expert who helps older adults and those with special needs throughout the country find the care they need. She specializes in dementia and other cognitive issues. A nationally recognized authority, she lectures frequently to caregivers, attorneys, financial advisors, and healthcare professionals. She is a former executive committee member of the Alzheimer's Association National Capital Area. Currently, she is an advisor to Second Act Financial Services, a division of Liberty Savings Bank, F.S.B. that specializes in resources for retirees; a senior associate editor of Vitality, Medicine & Engineering and the Journal of Aging Research and Lifestyle; and an advisor to the Brain Watch Coalition. An ardent patient advocate, Jodi helps people navigate the complicated, often convoluted system, identify what they need, and create an action plan. She is the co-author of *Brain Health As You Age* (Rowman and Littlefield 2018), a graduate of Brandeis University in Waltham, MA, and a former president of the Washington, D.C., area alumni association.